RECIPE FOR KICKING CANCER'S ASS

Brendan M. Lyons

Cover Artwork and Design:
Hallie R. Lyons

Dedicated to my dearest family and closest friends.

Recipe for Kicking Cancer's Ass

Ingredients:

Several liters of Normalcy

Humor sprinkled in to taste

Generous dollops of Family

Friends to add Texture

Zest of Personal and Family Experiences

Multiple Tablespoons of Reflection

Add in a liberal amount of Treats

Drip in Tears as needed

Fold in plenty of Documentation

Heaping helpings of Faith

Step 1: Mix it thoroughly, don't let it set, and eat generous helpings.

Step 2: Repeat Step 1 as much as possible, <u>PREFERABLY EVERY DAY</u>.

Author's Note:

This is not a book that guarantees a "cure" for Cancer. This book is very purposefully designed to make a hard distinction between a "cure" and "WINNING the battle with Cancer." Physical cures and mental WINS are two very different things and you will find out in the pages that follow exactly what I mean. I am in no way suggesting that you should not seek out professional medical advice and care and follow that protocol as prescribed with appropriate treatments and pharmaceutical interventions. Keep an open mind and really try to absorb the distinction that I am making in the words and "recipe" that I am going to share with you in the following pages for "WINNING the Battle with Cancer." I will use my own thoughts and philosophies to explain the ingredients but will support my positions with blog post entries that were authored throughout my wife Julie's battle with Cancer. The blog posts are italicized in the chapters that follow to make the distinction.

Additionally, you may note that I always capitalize the word "Cancer." This is a very conscious decision on my part, as Cancer, to me, is a living and breathing monster that demands proper noun status.

Prologue

Isn't it a great feeling to hear that a family member, a friend, a co-worker, an acquaintance (anyone really) has "WON or BEATEN their battle against Cancer"? On the flip side, think about what a downer it is when you hear someone "LOST their battle with Cancer." I have given a lot of thought to this and nothing irritates me more than to hear that someone LOST their battle. Who wants to exit this life as a "loser?" Not me. The unfortunate truth is that almost all of us have, or will have a very intimate encounter with this dreadful disease at some point in our lifetime. I am no exception to this rule.

In June of 2006, my youngest daughter was born and completed our family of five, two girls and a boy, and all very healthy. I had a great job with a great career path. My wife was a partner in her family's construction firm. We owned a home and two cars that were fully paid for. On top of that we had recently purchased a rental property as our first investment outside of our standard 401(k) plans. We had the world by the tail and things were really falling into place for Team Lyons and our bright future.

A couple years prior though we had a scare. There was a mole on my wife's back, right between the shoulder blades, that had been there ever since I had known her. You hear stories about irregular moles and skin Cancers and the *rare* melanoma. Skin Cancer is really no big deal because you just get it cut off and go on with life ... unless it is melanoma, but that is so rare and really shouldn't be considered. It rarely crosses anyone's mind. However, every time I knew my wife had a doctor checkup, I would be sure to remind her to have the doctor look at it. Each time she would do as she was asked. Each time the report would be the same. "It looks fine and you have nothing to worry about." OK then ... on with life!

Shortly after our son was born in 2003, she had one of her routine checkups. Again, we went through the process. Me reminding her to have that mole looked at and her insisting she would. When she returned home, she said the doctor had once again assured her it was fine, but told her since she asked about it each time she came in, he would refer her to a really good dermatologist who would remove it for her and they would never have to discuss it again. She quickly made the appointment and a few short weeks later she was at the dermatologist's office ready to have that thing scraped off and to never be of concern again.

She arrived at the office without a care in the world and ready to get this nuisance over with, as I am sure she had a full day planned. Julie never had a day where it wasn't jam packed with work, errands or kids' activities. She was never one to be idle. She carefully filled out the necessary paperwork required of a new patient and waited her turn. She was soon called back, weighed, and vitals were taken. All very healthy. Soon thereafter, the doctor arrived, and they quickly got to the topic at a hand ... the mole on her back, right between her shoulder blades. Almost immediately, the dermatologist said the mole was a problem and needed to come off that very visit sent to be biopsied. So, it was removed posthaste. A thorough full-body exam was conducted without any other areas of concern found by the doctor.

A week later, while driving home from picking up the kids, she received a call from the doctor's office with news about the biopsy. The results were in and had confirmed the mole was a melanoma. She pulled over to digest the news while the doctor herself on the other end of the line explained that they were working to get her in with a surgeon at The University of Texas M.D. Anderson Cancer Center, one of the premier Cancer treatment hospitals in the United States for more than a decade, and many argue that it is THE premier Cancer treatment hospital in the world. The plan would be to remove a larger margin around the mole site, test with nuclear dye to which lymph nodes that part of the body drained and remove them for biopsy as well.

This was scary news, but we were still naïve to how serious this situation we were facing would really be. Our biggest concern at the time was our 9-month-old son who was still breast feeding. Julie would be injected with a nuclear dye that would leach into breast milk; she was told to stop. We had never really introduced our son to a bottle at that point and he was not happy about the abrupt weaning process that was now being forced upon him. At this time this was Julie's biggest concern. She hated hearing him fuss because she could not provide him with what he really wanted. I look back on those days, scratching my head, as to how simple things were for us and how completely unaware of the gravity of our situation was in total.

The procedures were scheduled within the next two weeks and we headed to MDACC still not fully comprehending how serious this situation was. Our first trip to MDACC was simply a meet and greet with the surgical staff and the surgeon. The staff was very friendly and did everything necessary to put us at ease. They told us they had performed this procedure thousands upon thousands of times and we were in great hands. This doctor was one of the best in the world, which we found to be true of most of the doctors at this incredible facility.

The surgery was scheduled for a week or so later. We arrived ready to get this thing removed from both her body and our lives. We wanted to get back to our normal lives which included our children and our jobs.

The surgery went very smoothly and within a very short amount of time she was in the recovery room. All samples were sent to biopsy, and the doctor reported upon visual inspection that everything looked good. In fact, a few days later we were called back to the hospital and were given the good news that all samples were negative. This was a huge sigh of relief, but news we had expected to get all along. The surgeon said we were very lucky, and it appeared that we got it in time. However, there was a very small chance the mole had ulcerated and it could have penetrated the blood stream … no way to tell at present, but it was probably 10 percent chance or less. He told us we would be put on a six-month checkup schedule for the next 5 years. No big deal, we can handle that. Ten percent was just a small percentage. We were convinced we were done with it. After all, if you were told that you had a 10% chance to magically become a multi-millionaire in the next 12 months, how many of you are quitting your job tomorrow? I hope the answer is zero! We left the hospital in good spirits and ready to focus on getting on with life.

Fast forward two years to June 19 when our third child was born. Life was perfect. Our 6-year-old daughter and 3-year-old son were getting used to their new sister. Julie and I were getting used to parenting while being outnumbered by one! It was a big learning curve and things were hectic, but we were incredibly happy.

Later that summer, my parents organized a family reunion and rented a beach house in Galveston, TX. I had one uncle come in from Michigan, another uncle with his wife and my cousins from San Antonio, and my aunt along with the matriarch of our family, my grandmother whom we affectionately called "Gigi" had traveled in from California . We had a great time sharing meals, participating in beach activities and great family chatter. I also remember distinctly successfully getting my son potty trained on that trip. After only a few short months we were back to having only one child in diapers. What a win for us!

That was the last "normal" week in our life. We had no idea how that joy would turn to panic, fear, and despair so quickly.

The week after the conclusion of that family reunion, Julie was scheduled for her routine checkup. I didn't attend with her as all previous exams had shown nothing. It had been all good news and there was no reason to expect anything different this time. This would be her first full exam since the beginning of her pregnancy with our third child. Due to some of the tests they have to run, there is some concern as to the effects it may have on the pregnancy, so they forgo them altogether. Those exams still were fairly comprehensive, and the doctors had given her a clean bill of health each time. However, after this particular appointment, she called me at work with just a bit of apprehension in her voice. The tests had shown some abnormal markers and they were scheduling her for further tests. Ok, again no real concern on my part. She just had a baby, so maybe her body chemistry was still recovering. A normal mental reaction to try and justify the situation and avoid confronting any bad news. I was still on a high with the addition to our family.

The next test showed additional concerns especially around her liver. Finally, the doctors scheduled an invasive procedure to cut out a section of her body and do a comprehensive biopsy. The next several days we were on pins and needles waiting for a phone call that would free us from the prison of anxiety in which we were living. Every time the phone rang, we would jump and almost every time it was a work call or a friend wanting to see if we wanted to get together for dinner... normal "life" things.

Finally, that call came and it carried with it the worst news ever ... Stage 4 Melanoma.

I was at work that morning when she called. I had just hung up from a lengthy business call. I was taking my time consulting with an unemployed individual and desperately trying to find gainful employment again. Around 9 a.m. when my cell phone rang, it clearly displayed that Julie was on the other end of the call. I quickly, but politely, cut my business call short. She was in tears and explained to me what the doctor had said. My body went numb, my mouth went dry, and I immediately started to shake with the chills. This could not be. What did this mean? What was the prognosis? I was in a cloud and could not think clearly. I grabbed my keys and left the building for the 30 minute drive home, without telling anyone at work that I was leaving or what was going on. As I pulled out into the parking lot, I pulled out right in front of another vehicle causing him to slam on his brakes - narrowly avoiding a T-bone collision. I got a long horn honk and the finger, but that was the least of my concerns. I safely found the rest of the way home, where I found Julie sitting on the front porch swing, eyes red and swollen from tears, but not crying at present. She was slowly swinging while holding our baby in her arms who was sound asleep. I kissed her on the cheek and went inside to change out of my work clothes and get into something more comfortable.

I also took the opportunity to call the doctor to hear for myself what the diagnosis and prognosis was. As it turned out - not good. (Actually, this is a HUGE understatement, but I believe he was trying not to take all the hope from my spirit.) Very serious. Roughly a 15 percent chance of survival. I stopped him and told him specifically that I did not want a potential timeline relative to life expectancy. He told me to call him anytime if I had questions and gave me a direct number to use if needed. He closed the call by letting me know that MDACC Melanoma specialty unit would be in touch with us regarding a plan forward and chemo options very soon.

I joined my wife on the front porch swing and told her we were going to beat this thing -no matter what. We were going to WIN, I promised. She and I together - we were a team. She was not alone. Then we just cried for what seemed like hours. We got a call late that same afternoon from MDACC asking us if we could possibly come in that evening for some initial blood work and testing. Of course we could. We were not going to let any grass grow under our feet getting this battle started! But just making that commitment was tough. We had three small kids at home and no immediate plan for their care while we raced off to the hospital. We had not even told our parents what was going on. We had to get to get going. First, we called Julie's parents and broke the news, followed by a call to my parents. I have no recollection of those conversations what-so-ever. I don't remember how long the conversations lasted, how we communicated the news, their reactions ... nothing at all. I just know that the conversations happened quickly since we were short on time.

My parents, in their own state of shock, rushed over to watch the kids. We quickly left and made the drive to the Texas Medical Center in Houston where the vast and sprawling Cancer treatment and research facility resides. While we were at MDACC waiting for the tests, Julie asked what we should do for dinner ... ever the Mom making sure the kids were going to be fed and that we would take care of our basic needs. WHAT? ... talking about food??? I am crying my eyes out and have no appetite. Nevertheless, she placed a larger order of pizza for the kids, my parents, and us. The kid on the other end of the line had no idea of the situation of the person placing the order. Somehow, we got through the tests and left for the evening.

We arrived home and Julie had stopped crying and was her normal hostess self. She ate her pizza, shared some laughs and held a normal conversation with my parents. She also played with the kids. She had already started to kick

Cancer's ass. I ate nothing, cried in private as
not to upset the kids ... on the other hand, I was
letting Cancer kick my ass.

So begins the recipe for Kicking Cancer's Ass.

Chapter 1

Ingredient: Several liters of Normalcy

In a large mixing vat, add in several liters of normalcy. What do I mean by this? Life is full of mundane and normal tasks that you do every day to keep the household and your life running. Everything from getting up and getting dressed for the day, going to work, and managing your finances to doing household projects and maintenance. This Normalcy is what takes up most of the hours of your life. Don't give up on it! Get out of bed, get dressed, drink your morning coffee, go to work, call the A/C repairman to come service your unit, get your kids dressed and out the door for school, discipline them as necessary (they still need that as Cancer does not absolve you from raising your kids to be responsible adults) , start *and* finish projects, etc. You get the point. Life, at least until you exit this Earth, still goes on. Don't mentally give up and "die" if you or your loved one is diagnosed with the big "C."

As Cancer was still kicking my ass, I spent the next morning in my sleepwear sitting on the couch watching nothing that I can remember and crying nonstop. I can't even remember where the kids were at this time. Julie, on the other hand, came into the living room and very excitedly stated, "I am going to Home Depot. I need to buy some paint as I have been planning on painting Jackson's room and today is a good day to do that. Do you want to come with me?" Wait, um ... uhhh ... WHAT??? How can you even think about doing that at this point? You have stage 4 Cancer and you are thinking about going to Home Depot and painting a room? How can you even do that? Nevertheless, off she went to buy the paint she needed. She had the look she wanted all planned out in her head for our son's room. It was going to be a rugby – style - themed striped pattern around three of the walls and a large basketball key on the fourth wall using the same colors of light blue, orange and green.

She steadily, purposefully, and meticulously painted the room as if she were a professional painter. The first three walls took several hours as she had to do all the prep by laying down sheeting to protect the floors, properly tape the baseboards and tape the walls to produce the straight lines where the colors would transition. Guess what I was doing? Yep… sitting on the couch with the TV on, still not knowing what I was even watching and sobbing uncontrollably off and on.

Then she called to me … she needed help sketching out the basketball key. I played basketball all the way up through college and had spent several years officiating the sport at both high school and college levels. I was the resident expert on the dimensions, shape, markings, etc. I pulled myself together and went in and helped her. We took our time sketching it out to scale and making sure it looked perfect. When done, I stayed with her and picked up a brush and helped her paint that wall. The whole time I was working on this household project with my wife things were "normal." I didn't cry at all in those few hours as I was focused on doing something normal with Julie and improving something in our house for our family, in this case and more specifically, my son.

Below is a blog post I penned to demonstrate the importance of staying busy and doing the normal things in life that you would do had Cancer not invaded your life.

> *Keeping Busy – Tuesday, November 14, 2006*
>
> *Well it has been a few days since our last post, so I guess it is time for one (I don't want to disenfranchise any of our "ants" out there.)*
>
> NOTE - I will explain what I mean by "ants" in a later chapter
>
> *It has come to my attention that we have not been totally clear about Julie's current status since her last trip to the hospital. Those that we speak to regularly know that she was discharged a week ago last Friday. I have been told that some of you were not aware that she was discharged.*

Since then we have managed to keep ourselves very busy. Julie attended an all-day venture the day after her discharge (7 a.m. to 10 p.m.) with Hallie and the rest of their Daisy Scout troop up in Conroe. AMAZING. I will let her fill you in on the details of the episode so as not to steal her thunder.

The very next day we welcomed some good friends for a visit from the East Coast. We spent all day with them Sunday as they attended evening service with us and went to dinner. Julie ended up spending most of Monday running errands. Her friend was kind enough to travel around with her, catch up on things, and keep her company while her husband attended to some business in town and I got some work done in the home office. We all reconvened at our house for dinner and our friend made us a huge pan of lasagna and two tins worth of enchiladas for future fare!

The week was filled with its usual chaos of getting the

kids to and from school, trips to MDACC for blood work, soccer practice, homework and keeping up with our careers, which brought us to this past weekend where we exhausted ourselves once again ...

We had Hallie's last soccer game on Saturday, and it was by far her best game ever. She played forward in the second half and had many great kicks and she played goalie in the second half. She did not let one shot in, thanks to her many <u>spectacular</u> saves.

Hallie then filled the rest of her afternoon with a birthday party down the street while Julie did her best to entertain Kendall and Jack as I had to leave for a basketball game out of town (I am former High School and NCAA basketball official). An exhausting day for sure, so we took the next day off to relax right? NO ... I have Julie as a wife

....

She sent Jack in bright and early at 7 a.m. to wake me and Hallie up. If you don't know him, he is a bit of a spaz when he is excited so you can imagine the gentle awakening I received [sarcasm]. ***WAKE UP. WE HAVE TO GO TO THE FESTIBULL. I AM GONNA GETTA SWORD! COME ON. LET'S GO TO THE FESTIBULL. I WANNA SWORD.*** *Repeated many times over as he jumped like a wild man on the bed (kids just don't understand that you can't jump on their Dad's groins). That's right, Julie had planned us a day at the Texas Renaissance Festival, which is about an hour drive north of where we live. We got there about 10 a.m., spent a wad of cash and left about 2:30 for a reason I will explain in a minute. However, we had fun for about 2-5 bucks a pop every time I turned around (the sword for Jackson and the flower halo for Hallie were $15, however.)*

We had to race back home, because it was Sunday late afternoon which means time for the Daisy Scout Meeting of which Julie is the leader. So, on the way up to the festival, she cut up felt for the turkey beaks and gizzards to make turkeys as a craft she had in store for them. Jack and I on the other hand, got ourselves cleaned up and headed off to Sunday night service where my mom was kind enough to come along and keep us company. We all cratered in bed at about 8:30 that night!

*It sounds exhausting but it is what we need to do. By keeping busy we keep our mind off Cancer and enjoy our lives and family. If we idle, Cancer begins to dominate our life and consume us, which we **CAN NOT HAVE!** Truth is, Julie is the engine that makes this family go as she pushes us to stay active and get involved. Without her pushing us through this life*

In addition to keeping things normal on a day-to-day basis in terms of doing the regular things that life demands, it is imperative that you keep things normal for your children (assuming of course that you have children living at home while Cancer is living with you.)

When Julie was diagnosed with Cancer, we knew our lives would be a series of doctor's appointments, tests, inpatient stays, fatigue, exhaustion and a myriad of other obstacles. However, in the beginning we felt as though we could just use our large network of family and friends to cover the gaps. Some days my parents, affectionately known as "Mimi" and "Grandpa," or Julie's parents, "Nana" and "Poppa," would pick the kids up from school and take care of them while we were at the hospital. Other days, various friends who lived close to us wanted to help and would do so if they could. But we found that not only was this stressful on us always trying to make sure the kids transportation and other basic needs were being met it was also very stressful on the kids. Kids thrive on routine and Cancer had robbed them of the routine that they so desperately needed. They were dealing with a change in their parents' emotions, routines, and this foreign concept called "Cancer" and trying to process all of that. We noticed this immediately and knew we had to do something to fix this problem.

We started searching the internet and found several services that help identify individuals looking for full-time nanny positions. Even with the "match making systems" you must be careful and have some patience. We interviewed several via skype and narrowed it down to a few face-to-face interviews. We finally settled on one and spent time introducing her to the kids, explaining their routines, explaining our philosophies around raising our children in terms of how we instill discipline, praise, and other house rules. This seemed to be going well for the first few weeks and then the performance started to slip. Julie had made the decision that she would need to have a talk with her. The day the talk was to happen we waited and waited that morning for her to show up. She was late and not returning phone calls. I finally could not wait any longer and told Julie I needed to head to work. I got to the driveway to get into my truck and noticed our car seats with our house keys, and garage door opener resting in them. No note, but it was clear that she had abruptly resigned with no notice. This was a painful experience for both the kids and us as they had quickly taken to her. It was a jolt of rejection for us, but when you are fighting Cancer you have bigger things to concern yourself with than rejection and you must quickly regroup.

We contacted the service and they apologized profusely, cancelled her account and gave us a refund for our experience all while promising to help us make a match. Soon thereafter we were matched with a lovely and caring young lady by the name of Miss Ebony, as the kids would come to call her. My youngest who was just learning to talk when Miss Ebony came into our lives would soon take to calling her "Miss Abony," which we still laugh at today - 12 years later. Sometimes we still call her that just for a laugh. I wish I had a blog post to share with you on the introduction of Miss Ebony into our lives, but alas, I do not. She "worked" for us/me for roughly 5 years and has remained a close family friend to all of us. She is still very active in the lives of my children and she is very much part of our family.

One last example of keeping things normal for the family and children has to do with what is normal in the house. Julie and I always had dogs ever since we started dating. When I met Julie, she had a Chow Chow/Shar-pei mix by the name of Betsy, who could be a bit stubborn but had a wonderful temperament. She was always so patient with the kids, whether they were pulling on her ears, petting her gently (well - gently by toddler definitions) or dressing her up in their dress-up clothes. We also had a giant German Shepherd named Max, who also was very good with the kids while at the same time very protective of them. You had to convince Max that you meant no harm before he would even let you close to those kids.

Well 2007 was not a great year for us, as both Betsy and Max were aging. Long story short, Betsy, on a sunny morning "asked" to go outside, walked over to her favorite shade tree and quietly passed away. Two short months later, Max walked to the same tree, laid down and joined his sister in dog heaven. Yes, like I said, it was a tough year. But we had to keep things normal. We started looking at another dog soon after. You may think this is crazy with all the other things we had going on to add a new dog and all the responsibilities that come with that, but we felt it was important for "normalcy". So, the story went something like this taken from the following blog post.

> *Meet Sidney – Saturday, July 14, 2007*
>
> *Well we have a new addition to the family … Sidney! Julie and I have always had dogs ever since we have been together, and the kids have never known a home without a dog! When I met Julie in the summer of 1996, she had a dog named Betsy who was a mixed breed consisting of Chow Chow and Shar-pei and she was really a great and gentle dog. I had always wanted a dog as well growing up but for many reasons, never had one. So, I decided that when I was able, I was going to get one of my own*

as well. The weekend that Julie and I got engaged we decided to celebrate by adding another dog to our family. I found an advertisement in the newspaper advertising German Shepherds for a really low price and I had always liked that breed. The owner didn't have the AKC papers so he could not charge the higher breeder fees. Since we just wanted the dog for a pet and not a show piece, that didn't matter to us. We adopted Max. Well, last May, Betsy passed away after living a long life of about 13 years and Max passed away on July 2 after living 11+ years which is about average for a dog his size. So, for the first time in our kids' lives and the first time during our relationship we were "dogless."

After a trip to MDACC last week, we were both feeling a little heavy after a morning of dealing with the Big "C." It just so happens that the Houston SPCA is on the way home from the hospital so we thought we would stop in and see what they had to brighten our day. We looked at the really young puppies and they had a bunch of cute ones. But most were already adopted. There was another we really liked, but he was a male and Julie prefers females as they don't go around "marking" everything like males tend to want to do! So, we decided to see what was in the kennels for the larger dogs (besides, Julie has a big heart and feels sorry for the bigger dogs since everyone wants puppies.) This is where we found "Holly" who is a mix of an Australian Shepherd and something else (we don't know what!) She had such a cute little face and a gentle disposition. They allowed us to take her into one of the "get to know each other rooms" and after a few minutes Julie said "let's get her." So, we did. With the SPCA all pets must be fixed so we could not take her home right away. We told the kids over the weekend and since we determined that she was not all that attached to her name, that we would change it. Holly and Hallie just cannot exist in the same house!!! After a short search on the internet we decided on "Sidney." Hallie liked *it because it is a pretty girl's name and Jack liked it because there is a Power Ranger named Sidney. Thank goodness for that, because prior to that, Jack was insistent that we name the dog "Shiny Eye"... We have no idea where that came from or why he was set on that name. Sidney has settled in nicely and the kids absolutely LOVE playing with her. Unlike our last dogs, who were primarily outside dogs, Sidney is an inside dog and the real bonus. She came housebroken already! AWESOME. We could not be happier with her at this point. The biggest problem we have is keeping Kendall out of the dog food and from splashing in (or worse, dumping) the water bowl.*

More to come later. Thanks for checking in and all of the positive prayers and comments you guys leave us. They lift us up each day. We love you all (even those commenters we have never personally met ... thank you). Yay God.

Note - More to come on this last paragraph later but that it important to include it here.

Chapter 2

Ingredient: Humor Sprinkled in to Taste

I am sure almost everyone has heard the phrase "laughter is the best medicine" and there is plenty of science out there that shows that very specific chemicals are released in the brain and the body that have very beneficial effects. When one laughs the brain produces endorphins such as cortisol and epinephrine. Cortisol production is particularly important here as cortisol protects the body during times of crisis.

Just because you or your loved one has Cancer does not mean you are not allowed to laugh or find humor in things. Life is full of "Funny." Funny comes in many forms: embarrassing moments where you must laugh at yourself, comedy shows, TV or movies, jokes your friends or family tell you, social medial memes and many other forms and vehicles. Pay attention to them and get caught up in the "church giggles" or a big belly laugh when the funny fairy pays you a visit. Continue the family inside jokes and build more of them as life continues. Tell jokes or solicit jokes. Share an embarrassing story with your inner circle of friends. I promise you this will be a gut punch to Cancer as one of it's major goals is to steal your joy. People with no joy are already dying inside.

Most of my life I have been considered a bit of a smart ass and am fluent in sarcasm, but it has always been for the purpose of humor and never mean spirited. I am a jokester by heart and often tell people if you believe every fifth word I say you will probably get something that resembles accuracy or the truth! However, after Julie was diagnosed, my lighthearted spirit went away. I became stoic and somber. Something that I normally would find funny or crack a joke at was no longer humorous at all. I was content to just let the moment pass. I felt as though since I was dealing with such a horrific and terrifying disease, and my wife and best friend was fighting for her very life, nothing could be funny. How rude, insensitive, or selfish would it be to laugh at anything? It would be disrespectful if I ever joked or laughed at anything again. I had lost my ability to laugh and as such, I lost that natural medicine that would normally course through my body and give me the feeling of being alive. Those chemicals no longer circulated through me and my spirit for life itself was dying in the process. This went on for several weeks and my funny bone was in a severe state of necrosis, until as usual, Julie showed me that not only was it ok to make jokes and laugh, but I should because she was going to do just that.

A few weeks had passed since we were at MDACC for the initial tests and introduction to what our first treatment option was going to entail. We were waiting for the call back as to when her first chemo treatment would take place. On one particular morning, we were at a neighbor's house having a Bible study and praying for our family and Julie's medical/physical healing, when a phone call came. I stepped outside to take the call. It was MDACC and they were ready for us. They had a spot available that day and we needed to get down there as soon as possible for her first chemo treatment. Needless to say, excitement and fear simultaneously coursed through our bodies. Excitement as we could finally get on with medically attacking the tumors in her body and hopefully make progress toward physical healing, but fear in the thought of chemotherapy, and the toll it would take on her body. Would she lose her hair and take on the appearance of Cancer? Would she be nauseous all the time? Would she be overly fatigued and want to sleep all the time? Nonetheless, we made quick arrangements for the kids and jumped in the car and made the ever ominous and never changing 45-minute drive.

If you have never been to The University of Texas M.D. Anderson Cancer Center, that is a very good thing, but if you ever need it, there is no better place to be. The biggest problem is that the facility is a massive and sprawling system of buildings connected by skybridges, tunnels, hallways etc. However, every staff member and volunteer is supremely trained to get you where you need to go, and do so in a friendly way. They know that no matter what is going on in their day, or how bad their day is personally, the people they are serving are having some of the worst days of their lives. We finally figured out the parking situation and through the help of several staff members we were guided to the area that was going to administer our chemo. We had no idea what to expect. After some preliminary paperwork and questions, we were led through some double doors that revealed hallways with standard-looking hospital rooms on either side. We were let into one room with a beautiful view of the medical center towers and you could see a bit of the Rice University campus in the distance. We were scared. No idea what to expect or how this would work. It was all happening so fast but not fast enough all at the same time.

The nurse finally entered the room. I will let the blog post below describe what happened next in detail.

Humor IS Medicinal –
Thursday, October 12, 2006

In the last couple of weeks, humor has almost been non-existent in our lives, for obvious reasons. Which, if you know me at all, is hard to fathom as I try and inject humor in almost everything I do. I like to give people some good-natured ribbing and receive some in return. I like to play harmless practical jokes on people and friends and in return they have played many on me. I like to tell a good joke and hear one in return. But mostly, I like to tell and hear true stories that have an inherent laugh contained within.

Humor and wit are how I break the ice when I meet new people. It is what I use to bring a stressful business, family, officiating, or personal situation back to a manageable level. It helps remind me and those around me not to take everything in life so seriously.

When we received "the news" a couple of weeks ago, however, I didn't feel as though I would ever laugh again. When you receive news of that nature your shoulders slump, you lose the "pep in your step" and you wonder how you will get through the next day, hour, or even minute. It is hard to imagine anything that will lift the spirits to the point of laughter or even smile.

Julie continues to amaze me as she takes on this fight. Within a couple of days, she dug in her heels for this battle and basically returned to her old self, (painting the kid's rooms, running errands, going on her morning jogs, etc.) as if we weren't carrying this albatross around our collective necks. She was even sharing a smile and laugh when the moment struck her. I, on the other hand, was completely paralyzed and walking around in a foggy haze.

A shining example of this spirit is evidenced in this true story ...

This past Monday was Julie's first chemo treatment. The possible side effects of the treatment are outlined in our paperwork and are roughly two pages long. They all sound awful and, in many cases, extremely painful. So, to say the least, we were both on edge and anxiety was HIGH. This anxiety was only heightened when they called our name and took us back to the "treatment rooms." My anxiety was to the point that I was lightheaded and could feel my heart racing. Looking around the rooms you could see people laying in their beds with IVs and bags upon bags of chemicals being infused into their bodies. Outwardly, I knew I had to be strong for Julie, however, on the inside, my body was generating its own chemotherapy and producing horrible side effects. They checked her in, once again taking note of her height, weight, temperature, blood pressure and pulse. Once complete, they escorted us to our room where we waited for the nurse to come in and start her IVs that would administer the chemo drip. Of course, this took some time as well, which allowed tensions to build further. When the nurse came in to start, she greeted us with the standard, "Hello. How are you?" For most, this is an automated greeting that is empty and generally followed by an equally empty and automated response of "Fine. How are you?" and the dialogue goes from there. In the instant before Julie responded, several thoughts raced *through my mind. The responses that went through my head where along the lines of, "What do you think? We are pretty Sh*tty right now. We have this insidious disease and the only way to get rid of it is coming here for you to stick her with needles and fill her body with poison to kill off the Cancer cells blah, blah, blah. How are you doing? Pretty good I would guess [sarcasm]!" Julie, however, responded rather flippantly and nonchalant (in fact she used no chalant what-so-ever; Credit to Lou Fertle for that expression), "Well ... I got a bit of the Cancer today." As if she was reporting to the nurse, "Well, I scraped my knee and would like a Band-Aid." The nurse (as I) were all first shocked by the response. However, a few moments later we were ALL IN LAUGHTER. You had to be there, but it truly was great and broke the tension. I don't care who ya are ... that's funny right there.*

*Within a week and a half, I had forgotten what it felt like to laugh and, in that case, it **truly was the best medicine for both of us.***

Julie … thanks for reminding me how to laugh and smile and facilitating that process. I LOVE YOU AND THAT LOVE GROWS EACH DAY!

Now if you will indulge me for just a minute. I don't want this book to be all about blog posts. I want there to be a lot of content and thought supporting why I think these ingredients are important. I am trying to limit most chapters to one blog post to drive home the point and support my position. However, I mentioned that you should "Sprinkle in Humor to taste," and for it to taste really good to me I need a lot of Humor, so I am going to OVER sprinkle for my particular taste.

I want to share this post that I wrote late at-night but for it to make sense I need to provide you with some context. I authored this post around 2 in the morning (you will see why in a minute). We were having a weeklong, inpatient, chemo treatment - which was always hard. The kids could only come for short visits, we were essentially confined to a hospital room as Julie was hooked up to several lines and just getting to the bathroom was an act of Congress.

Additionally, this was just before the time of Netflix streaming and all the other on-demand programming that is available today. I used to purposefully turn on the daytime programming of Maury Povich, Jerry Springer and Judge Judy just to irritate her! I should note that while she despised that programing it was playful irritation as she knew what I was up to. Julie was peacefully sleeping in her bed and I was tossing and turning on the contraption that was available for the spouse, partner or close family member to spend the night with their loved one. The post I authored tells it best so I will let it speak for itself.

A Proper Tribute to the Bouch - Thursday, December 21, 2006

Well Julie gave it the old college try in her earlier post to introduce the Army to the "Bouch." However, due to her chemo brain and the simple fact that she has not logged any time on this fine piece of engineered furniture she fell well short in giving it its proper due!

As previously mentioned, it has been appropriately named as the Bouch by a friend of mine. The word is simply derived by combining the words "bed" and "couch." Now some might say that it is incorrectly named

*and should be called a "Bair"
due to the fact that when it is
transformed to its most
upright position, it resembles
more of a chair than an actual
couch. However, as the
resident expert on Bouches, I
will vehemently argue against
this position. Why you ask?
Because anyone who has spent
as many hours on this thing, in
all of its various positions (it is
a very versatile piece of
furniture as I will demonstrate
later) will note the word 'ouch'
contained within is just as
important a reference as the
bed and the couch!*

*Now being the father of three
young children, I have had
many experiences with
bouches in the recent past so
my memory on their comfort
level and designs is quite fresh.
I have now spent extensive
time on 3 different bouch
designs and I can say without a
doubt that all are
HORRENDOUS!*

*However, there is a difference
in comfort level and the one
here at MDACC is the best.
Please let's keep this in context
... NONE OF THEM ARE*

COMFORTABLE BY ANY STRETCH OF THE IMAGINATION!!! But, in all fairness, it is the best of the three. Hallie was born in Clear Lake Regional and its bouch comes in second place. So which hospital has the worst BLBR (Brendan Lyons Bouch Rating)? The booby prize goes to Memorial Hermann Hospital in Memorial City where my son Jackson and newest daughter, Kendall were born, and it is a distant third on the BLBR. I don't have a picture of the Clear Lake Bouch, but I do have one of the Memorial Herman bouch. Its design is such that you have to precariously balance the back cushions (when it is in couch formation) on a narrow extension that slides out when one of the arms is pulled out from the body of the unit. The cushions never stay in place and you are lucky to only have to reposition them four times throughout one night of un-restful slumber. To make matters worse, since the arm is still at the end when it is pulled out, tall people (I am 6'4") have to suffer through sleeping in somewhat of a quasi-fetal position that does not facilitate the cushions staying in place whatsoever!

Now, Bouches do ALWAYS have a few commonalities other than they are all uncomfortable. First and foremost, they always are upholstered with the lowest grade vinyl on the market. Second, they all have HIDEOUS colors and patterns. Nothing like you would ever find on any other piece of furniture in the world! I have come to the conclusion that all vinyl fabric that comes out of the dye process with a major defect or a color experiment that came out horribly wrong, immediately gets sent out to the Bouch manufacturers and it becomes a win, win. The vinyl producers get to unload this horrible abomination of color and patterns, and the Bouch makers get cheap coverings which keeps the cost down when the hospitals buy in bulk. The only loser is the end user, which is generally the caregiver in the situation. And third, they are always in some form of disrepair. Sometimes the slides *stick, the hydraulics are shot (I actually fell through one last time when I sat down on the end pull out module) or (in most cases) the vinyl is ripped/torn in one or more places.*

Now why I ask, are Bouches used in hospitals? There is no other place in America where you will find a Bouch ... not even prisons. Not even prison I said, where you would think they would be ideal. A place for our country's vermin to sit and sleep without purchasing two different pieces. Perhaps it was tried at one point, but I am sure that the concept was abandoned as it would not pass the "cruel and unusual punishment" litmus test.

Are caregivers not as important to the whole wellness process as the patient themselves? The usage of the bouch, in my opinion would suggest just that. But we all know that caregivers are an integral part of the process to the loved ones return to health. In this country we have organizations that look out for the ethical treatment and wellbeing of prisoners, patients, the elderly, the youth, the unborn. Heck, there is a huge organization that concern themselves with the ethical treatment of animals (PETA). I am not questioning that these are not worthy endeavors, buy why not CAREGIVERS?!?! I believe I may start a movement to address the ethical treatment of caregivers ... People for the Ethical Treatment of Caregivers Organization (PETCO) ... WAIT THAT WON'T WORK EITHER. People will be contacting me all the time to help them with their pet supplies. I am no expert on litter boxes or bird cages! I will have to come up with something better. (In the blog I included pictures of all the various bouch formations)

Obligatory Julie update ... Nothing new to report on day 3. Her body is tolerating the treatment quite well still. Her hair is really starting to thin, but that is just cosmetic and not painful. All vitals are in good order and the only major side effect seems to be the fatigue. YAY GOD!!!

Well I will sign off now, and I hope you enjoyed my twisted sense of humor. As I look at the clock, it is now well past 2 in the morning. A critical component to falling asleep on the Bouch is that you have to be EXHAUSTED, otherwise you will toss and turn on the creaking vinyl for hour,s prolonging your agony! After authoring this piece of satire, I have now reached exhaustion. Goodnight to all and I hope that you all rest well on your double/queen/king pillow-top mattresses ... sigh!!!

Love to the Army, until next time ...

Chapter 3

Ingredient: Generous dollops of Family

Pride gets in the way of a lot of things. Many of us want to handle our problems on our own, especially for men in the culture of machismo that we live. However, Cancer is a Goliath and very few of us are David. It is imperative that you set pride aside and leverage family for as much assistance as necessary. Remember, they are your blood and, in most cases, these are the people in your life that will stick with you through thick and thin. To be clear, when you are battling Cancer, you are definitely in the "thin". It matters not if you are mastering the world, failing miserably, solving world problems or making horrible errors in judgment. These are the people that love you unconditionally and want to help. They want, and in most cases need, to be part of the solution. Let them. Think if the shoe were on the other foot and one of your family members was in your shoes and continually stiff armed you on your offers to get involved and help. Would this turn into a WIN? I guarantee that it would not make you feel good. Let them in and let them help. This is therapy for them as well. Now don't get me wrong, boundaries must be established and what their help will consist of needs to be clearly defined. Remember the first ingredient of Normalcy. You don't want them interjecting so much that your normalcy dilutes in the vat. It will compromise the taste of the WIN in the end. However, there are so many things that need to be done when you are waging war against Cancer that the extra soldiers on the battlefield will be needed and welcomed.

I highly recommend having a close family member with an attention to detail to attend most, if not all, doctor appointments where the topics might include treatment options, results, next steps, etc. This is because you and your loved one are going to react very emotionally to most of the news that is given. This could be positive emotions when results are favorable or negative emotions when the expected results are not realized. When you are emotional it is natural not to catch all the necessary details and information that is provided. It is helpful to have someone close to you that can listen and take good notes for you so that you can review later and make prudent choices. It is important to take an active role in your own medical care in many cases and it is good to have someone take these notes and research your medical paths forward yourself. Today there is a vast amount of technical and medical information available online and through networking. Let family assist with this aspect as well. The more information you have the better your chances of success become, regardless of prognosis. Think of it in terms of adding ammunitions and ordinance to your bunkers for the battles that will be coming.

Family (and later we can discuss friends) can also assist with some financial necessities as well. Cancer is expensive and not all things are covered by insurance. Consider parking fees, as M.D. Anderson Cancer Center (and other medical facilities around the country) is not cheap and can add up. Family is also useful for taking the occasional dinner order as sometimes treatments take so long, and you are so exhausted that this is really the only option. Eating out is far more expensive than cooking for yourself. If you order out too many times you can find yourself behind on your monthly budgeting quickly. Managing finances and bills is also a good task to delegate, if you are comfortable doing so. It can all get away from you very quickly and cause significant headaches getting utilities restored, credit cards reactivated, or credit back to a reasonable score.

Again, you have to be careful that you don't outsource everything as you don't want to compromise your key ingredient of Normalcy. But you have an added component in your life called Cancer that is going to demand a lot of your time and attention. Maintenance of your assets still needs to be handled. Sometimes it is taking your car to get its oil changed or tires rotated while you are in for a weeklong inpatient treatment. Other times the A/C at your home or another appliance needs to be serviced and there is no way for you to be there to meet the serviceman. This is yet another place where family can come help and even save the day. Family is your best source of support in these situations as they often have keys to your home and sometimes vehicles, but the only other people that are going to care as much about maintaining the value of your assets as much as you, is your family.

But the most basic, yet I would argue the most fundamental function family can provide, is love and support. Sometimes you just need someone who can listen with no agenda to your thoughts and fears; hug and hold you when that is all that you want. Even as an adult you WILL need this, trust me. You will need them so that you can just vent if that is truly what you need to do. Conversely, it is so helpful to have someone there to possibly even celebrate in the smallest piece of good news. They can help provide discussion on topics outside of Cancer. Trust me you will get sick of talking about Cancer nonstop and when you are at MDACC or a similar facility you are surrounded by people talking about nothing else but that subject. Doctors and nurses passing through the halls, family and friends of other patients talking on cell phones giving their network the latest update. The talk around you will become CANCER, CANCER AND MORE CANCER. Having family around you can give you something other than Cancer to talk about such as world events, sports, arts and crafts and other lighter topics. Trust me, you will need this.

GiGi – Wednesday, November 01, 2006

I am long overdue to dedicate a post to this woman … My paternal grandmother Gigi …

This lady goes by several different names; Mom, Grandma and over the last couple of years GiGi (shortened version of Great Grandma) by my three wonderful children.

She is my paternal grandmother and one of the most amazing people one could ever meet. She is very much like a fine wine ... she just gets better with age!

*She currently lives with my aunt in Walnut Creek, CA. However, as she will often tell you, she is not tied to anything and she just travels to wherever she is needed. Well, it just so happened that we **<u>NEEDED</u>** her here in Houston. The day we received the news of Julie's diagnosis, she got on the phone, booked herself a ticket on the next flight out and arrived in Houston late that same evening. She has been staying with us ever since, with a few periodic breaks over weekends, etc. out at my parent's house. And let me tell you what a help she has been.*

She does all kinds of things around the house and most of it is stuff that we intend to do but she beats us to it. (e.g. folding laundry, emptying the dishwasher, fixing kids periodic snacks, etc.) But by far and away, her favorite chore is taking care of baby Kendall.

She lives for taking care of this baby. Usually, the third child in a family has some pretty well-developed lungs due to the fact that they have to cry and be heard to get attention. Not baby Kendall! GiGi is right there to scoop her up at the first sign of agitation or distress on her part. Bottles are always clean and prepared, diapers are changed on the regular, and if those are not the issue, they head out to the front porch swing to enjoy the fall weather and the light swinging motion.

Having her here is great for us, as it helps us keep the many medical appointments we have as well as allowing us to keep up with our careers even though on a somewhat more limited basis. Thanks for being who you are to us Grandma

*and for everything that you do
to help us.*

<u>WE LOVE YOU!!!</u>

Chapter 4

Ingredient: Friends to A\add Texture

Similar to family, friends are the next best thing. In fact, many of you have friends that are just like family. I have a circle of friends that makes it a point of meeting up at least once a year. In fact, this gathering was started by Julie on July 4, 1996. It is a river floating trip in central Texas on the Frio River. We have been going on this trip for more than 25 years now. This group of friends has come to call ourselves "handpicked family." You don't always get to pick your family, but you always get to pick your friends.

Friends play a very a similar, yet different role in your life when your family is battling Cancer. It is unlikely that they can be there to support you as much as your family can as they have their own lives they still need to lead. They have jobs and careers to focus on, kids to tend to and get to and from school, and all sorts of extracurricular activities. They have their own problems that need to be addressed, whether they be other relationships or needs of their significant others, financial obligations, job stressors , family issues of their own etc. However, despite all of this, they are your friends and want to play a role in kicking Cancer's ass in whatever capacity that they can.

Friends are also excellent at coordinating the timing of food deliveries that will come from all sorts of other friends - both close friends and those that know you through church, children's athletics, Scouting and the like. If not carefully planned and coordinated, you are going to end up with seven casseroles, nine pans of lasagna, seventeen pounds of salad (both traditional and fruit), and thirty four loaves of garlic bread, and if you are lucky, only 10 cakes and 12 pies on any given night. This is true especially early in the process. Let a friend or two spearhead that operation and space things out to a manageable level so that things don't go to waste. Trust me, it doesn't feel good when you know people have gone out of their way to help you and you know their efforts are going to go to waste.

Another often overlooked need friends can provide is just someone to hang out with and talk to. Talk about what is going on in your life. The regular stuff, the medical stuff, world events and jokes. Friends are generally the best for just listening and making you feel "normal." Let's be honest, family is great in most cases, but friends are the ones we generally seek out to go have a good time. Maybe it is just to hang out and watch a good game, a movie or binge watch a Netflix original series. Perhaps you just want to chat over a glass of wine or your favorite beverage of choice. Invite them over as they would probably welcome the opportunity to come over. Remember "normalcy?" You would probably do that had Cancer not invited itself over first, so keep inviting friends over as well. Cancer hates company, so do it if for no other reason just to piss it off! But be sure to invite them, since many times they purposely stay away thinking it is best to give you some space and they don't want to impose or feel like they are inviting themselves.

Social media is also a powerful tool to engage friends and build new friends along the way as they jump on the team to help you beat Cancer. When Julie was battling her Cancer, social media was in its infancy. Facebook wasn't even a real thing yet! But blogs were taking off and we decided to leverage this tool for two purposes. We were growing very tired of repeating the latest medical updates, progresses, regresses, next steps and all the other questions that your family and friends are wanting to know. A blog was perfect for this. We could post our updates once and anyone who cared to see the latest news could log in and catch up on their own time. We only had to take the time to update once each time there was something new to report.

But the blog had another positive effect that we did not count on - nor did we even consider. It had the power of growing our network of supporters. Almost every day, a new person would log in and leave us a comment in addition to our normal family and core group of friends that would always leave comments. Science has proven that there are certain chemicals that are released in the brain that almost produce a "high like" sensation when someone "likes" or comments on your social media. In today's world, this is both good and bad. Good, in that people can keep up with each other and stay in contact in this very busy world but bad in that it can become an addiction and we lose the ability to participate in the real world and enjoy life in the moment that is right in front of us. However, in this case the blog was truly a blessing for us. Whenever we logged back on to a recent post and saw the comment count rise, a rush of excitement, anticipation and happiness coursed through our veins which was always welcome. We enjoyed seeing who logged in to check on us and we always drew encouragement from every comment no matter how brief. Those little boosts of positive energy that we received with each comment left was very therapeutic. It was definitely a tool to leverage our friends and involve them by the masses to kick Julie's Cancer right in the ass.

Lastly, as mentioned earlier, Cancer is a very expensive financial proposition and sometimes family can only do so much. Luckily for us, we had a good medical plan and Julie had the foresight to purchase a supplemental insurance plan that covered a Cancer diagnosis which helped greatly, and I would say that we had a solid financial situation. We were not "rich" by any stretch of the imagination, but we were doing oOK. Even so, there are so many costs that come that are not addressed by any of the above-mentioned coverages. Again, we were lucky enough to live in the same city as MDACC which I previously said, is a premier institution for treating Cancer patients. However, many are not as fortunate. Many must travel, which includes gasoline, oil, tires, maintenance costs and/ or air travel, rental cars, hotels, meals, and the list goes on. Incidentally, we found ourselves in a position, which I will mention later, where we had to fly to Dallas and back one day per week. This is expensive. The point of all of this is, don't be so prideful that you don't allow friends who want to help, help cover costs that would otherwise put a financial burden on you and cause even more stress. Dealing with Cancer is stressful enough. I am not saying go out and specifically ask for money, but if a friend offers to assist financially - or in some cases, insists on it - don't be afraid to accept. In many cases this is the only way they can help you out as they live too far away, travel consistently for work or have so much going on in their own lives that it takes all their free time just to keep their own lives on track. Additionally, when you are in a better place and this ordeal is behind you, you can always choose to pay them back or better yet, pay it forward. That way you don't have to feel like you are accepting handouts and let your pride get in the way of receiving the help you can certainly use during this critical time in your lives.

It takes an army to beat Cancer and every soldier has their role. Your closest friend(s) can be the Generals that rally the troops and assign the roles to flank the enemy and steadily show that no matter how hard it tries, it cannot steal your joy. It cannot terrorize you to the point you stop living your life and engaging in life's moments in real time.

I share this post to provide a shining example of what I'm talking about:

treatment. We did not know just yet what time we needed to be there as they were to call back with that information. We decided to go ahead and go to the Bible study while we waited for the return call. However, I needed to make a few phone calls to family to finalize arrangements for the kids, work and the rest of our obligations since we had not planned on being at the hospital for the day.

This is when I saw "the sign." As I was speaking on the phone I was looking down at the sidewalk and noticed a worm that had recently died (I know this because it was not baked to a crisp yet in the hot Houston sun). OK, not that interesting but it gets better. This worm was being dragged all the way across the sidewalk by an army of ants. I watched it all the way as they got to the edge of the sidewalk and then dropped off into the grass and then into the newly developed ant hill where I can only imagine that the colony devoured it. The worm was several times the size and weight of each one of those ants and there is no way one or two of those ants could have accomplished that feat. However, working together as an "army" it was accomplished rather swiftly and efficiently.

Here is the analogy that I believe God was trying to show me ... the worm represents the Cancer that has become an UNINVITED GUEST in Julie's body. The ants represent Julie, me, family, friends, colleagues and the network of people that have grown from this nucleus by word of mouth, prayer list, etc. Julie and I could not move this "worm" on our own. However, I believe that God has sent me a message that he hears us and together with our "army" praying with us and God performing his miracles, Julie will WIN her battle with Cancer and we will devour this worm!

This is not a pretty example, but I have always said that if I get in a fight with something bigger than me, I don't plan to fight fair! I'm calling in ALL my Friends.

Therefore, please keep the positive thoughts and prayers coming our way and leave us a note. This blog has only been active for a few days and we are overwhelmed at the outpouring of support thus far. It is very humbling, and all of your comments are very therapeutic to us and our families.

With Love and Gratitude,

Brendan

Chapter 5

Ingredient: Zest of Personal and Family Experiences

As I mentioned earlier, it is important to keep doing things and having experiences. Recall our trip to the Texas Renaissance Festival? I can still look back on that day with my wife and three kids and while I don't remember everything, I do have a snapshot memory of buying a big bag of apples and feeding them to the elephants (one of the attractions was elephant rides) as passengers were loading and unloading. The squeals, giggles and amazement of my young children watching the elephants gently reach out to them with their trunks, deftly grab the apples from their tiny hands, swing it into their mouth and devouring them whole was worth every penny spent that day. I get a little smile on my face every time I think of that moment we shared as a family.

Another time, the weekend was upon us and we really didn't have much planned. So, as we were apt to do before we had kids, we made an impromptu plan to head to San Antonio for the weekend and take the kids to Sea World. (Now I know I may lose a few of you here given the press that Sea World has gotten in recent years post release of the documentary "Black Fish." Truth be told, I am not a fan at this point and will not likely ever visit this particular park again.) However, I do look back on that trip during this period of our lives and it gives me a warm feeling inside. The kids loved feeding fish to the pool of Bottled-Nosed Dolphins and laughing at the silly antics at the Sea Lion and Walrus show. The look of awe and amazement as they watched Shamu launch its massive body into the air and return to the tank with a massive splash. This was all fun for us parents to see the look of wonderment and joy in our childrens" eyes. However, strangely enough that is not the most vivid memory I hold onto from that trip. At one point in the day we took a break from the shows and went to the "carnival" part of the theme park. I absolutely HATE these things as you shell out dollar after dollar, playing games that are rigged in the "house's" favor in an effort to win cheap prizes. There are not many things I enjoy more than spending 25 dollars trying to win a small stuffed animal that is worth roughly 79 cents. (Remember when I said I was fluent in sarcasm? I wasn't lying about that.) While we were at the carnival, Jackson spotted a fishing game that he wanted to play since (a) he liked fishing, and (b) the prize was a small green dragon stuffed animal. Jack was a collector of stuffed animals. He had so many in fact that I have no idea how he even slept in his own bed. What 4-year-old boy would not want to add a green dragon stuffed animal to his bed and overall collection? I stood off to the back both fuming at the amount of money we were spending on this thing but also, smiling watching both he and his mother's determination to get the job done. I took a picture of their efforts and was both relieved and proud when they finally found success! Jackson is now 16 years old and has parted with most of his stuffed animals (thank goodness). However, the green dragon still exists and sits on the nightstand dutifully watching over him as he sleeps each night.

One of the "blessings" that came from our battle with Cancer was a trip to Switzerland to try another medical attack on the disease. When she was first diagnosed, we were given options which many patients are given at the onset of their medical treatment. We were told that there was a clinical trial that she was eligible to participate in now if she so chose. However, if she started with the standard of treatment, this particular trial option would be off the table. Therefore, we decided to go with the trial. After a few administrations of this protocol, scans revealed that it was not having the desired effect in shrinking her tumors. We then went to the standard of treatment, which again produced the same results ... no positive effects. In fact, tumors were growing, and they were popping up elsewhere. We were then told by our doctor at MDACC that there was another trial underway at Baylor Medical center in Dallas (this is why I mentioned earlier where financial assistance from family and friends came in handy). We did this for a couple of months traveling to and from Dallas from Houston every Wednesday. We had friends chip in and pay for our airfare. A co-worker made arrangements with a car rental company to comp all of our rentals and a dear friend of Julie's in Dallas put us up in her house to cover sleeping accommodations when needed (most trips were up and back in one day).

Once again, we hit a brick wall in terms of medical success. We returned to our primary oncologist at MDACC and once again he offered another idea. There was a standard of treatment available in Australia and a few countries in Europe but was not approved (at the time and still don't know if it is yet) by the FDA in the United States. He could match us up with a doctor over there, have them assess her, prescribe the chemotherapy regimen, pick it up there and travel back to the states with it. As long as it was prescribed by a medical doctor in a country that had it approved as standard treatment protocol, MDACC could administer it to her at their facility in Houston ... I know, I know, isn't government helpful sometimes!

In all actuality, this was truly a blessing for us. My parents happened to have a very close friend who lived just outside of Geneva, Switzerland, only a 45-minute drive to Lausanne, where there was a hospital and a doctor who was familiar with our oncologist at MDACC. A phone call from him and she agreed to meet with us. We had a place to stay at no cost and a friend who covered our flight costs in conjunction with the help of some frequent flier miles I had amassed through business travel. Since we were already going to be over there, and outside of having Cancer in her body, Julie felt relatively healthy (which sounds strange to say). We decided to stay there for roughly a month and have the first few cycles administered there and enjoy a fabulous European vacation as a family at the expense of Cancer. While we were there, we did so many things together that I look back on and cherish those memories. No one can ever steal the memories of those times from me. The memories I have of that magical time with my wife and kids in Switzerland are priceless to me. Money and things are replaceable. Experiences and memories are irreplaceable. Luckily, if you follow this recipe for Kicking Cancer's ass, they could become an impenetrable vault that can never be lost or stolen.

During this trip and in between treatments we traveled around Geneva like locals just exploring the city. We took several road trips through the southern part of France where we dined on fine cheeses paired with the perfect wine (not the kids ... they focused on hot chocolate and crème puffs of course), crepes infused with Grand Marnier and other wonderful French cuisine. We traveled to the German part of Switzerland up to Interlaken and took in the beautiful scenery there by taking a tram to the top of one of the mountains. We traveled around Lake Geneva on a paddle wheeler, riding in the first-class section, even though we only bought economy tickets (I think it is OK to admit that now as the statute of limitations has surely expired). We took a roadie into the Italian part of Switzerland to get a taste of the culture for that region and hiked to some of the glaciers. We took many pictures which are near and dear to me but are a distant second to the pictures that were taken in my brain of those experiences. Lastly, since we were approaching our 10-year anniversary together, our hosts decided to send us on a weekend excursion to Rome - sans kids. A romantic getaway for the two of us in Rome … Take that Cancer … do you really think you are WINNING despite your tumors? GO TO HELL, we are living our best lives as if you are not even there! While in Rome, we stayed at the gorgeous hotel Michelangelo just outside the gates of the Vatican. We took a guided tour of the Vatican and the Sistine Chapel and then we hiked, in the blazing hot summer that exists in Rome, all over the city to see the Colosseum, the Trevi Fountain, the Pantheon and some of the major plazas in the city. We ate gelato in the sun and had a magnificent anniversary dinner at Alfredo's … the birthplace of the Alfredo Sauce.

In addition to all these excursions, we had plenty of restful days at our friend's home in Coppet. We sat by their pool drinking Nescafe while the kids jumped and played in the backyard pool. Our hosts and Hallie did "bomba" after "bomba" (our hosts were Spanish and bomba translates to cannonball). From their house on a clear day we had a wonderful view of Mount Blanc. We did a lot of blogging from this spot in addition to just living our lives, but having conversations with each other, sharing our fears, our happiness and all the other things that couples and families do on a normal day.

Below is one of my favorite blog posts from our trip to Switzerland to fully explain how special this ingredient was to us in our battle:

A Trip into the Alps – Saturday, August 4, 2007

The weather cooperated with us, for the most part yesterday. It was sunny but the sky still had a lot of clouds. We decided that we were going to go for it and head to Chamonix, France to see the Les Bossons Glacier and Mont Blanc, which is the highest mountain in Western Europe. On a clear day you can see the capped peak from our host's backyard.

The mountain itself is in France and is roughly an hour or so drive through the alpine countryside. Along the way we were treated to beautiful views of Jet d'Eau in Geneva which can be seen for miles (or kilometers as they use here), jagged mountain peaks and glacial waterfalls. Spectacular to say the least. We then arrived in Chamonix and our breath was taken away. It was literally like walking through a postcard! The sidewalk cafes were abundant, ice cream shops and unfortunately for parents ... souvenir shops on every corner. Yes, we buckled under the pressure. Jack got a new monster truck (ironically, it is what he wished for on his torch for National Day [this is a holiday in Switzerland discussed in a separate blog post]) and Hallie got a chunk of amethyst crystals from the mountain.

One of the more interesting sites we saw was actually on (or should I say "IN") the river through town. For all the Texan Tubers out there ... this is what I would call "Extreme Tubing" ... You have to wear a helmet and wetsuit that must be several millimeters thick to prevent hypothermia in the water. The current is unbelievably fast and I doubt there is much concern about places you might have to "get up and walk." The only thing I can tell that they don't do right is bring along a tube to hold the ice chest full of beer and a river radio to blast the Corey Morrow tunes!!!

We made our way to Montenvers Train to head up the mountain to get a better view of the mountains and the valley that Chamonix rests within, as well as the Glacier that is carving its way through the mountains. It's about a 20-minute ride up the mountain that contains majestic view after majestic view … We just could not stop taking pictures.

Once on top of the mountain, we took a small hike with the kids down to the glacier (amazing that despite her Cancer and treatments she was still strong enough to hike mountains … again another giant "FU" to Cancer). We were a little concerned that the kids would have a hard time making the climb back up as it was very steep and of course the mountain air is a whole lot thinner than what we are used to at sea level back home! I had visions of giving Jack a ride on my shoulders back up most of the incline. However, to our surprise, the kids bounded right back up the trail and it was mom and dad who were left in the dust huffing and puffing and gasping for oxygen.

I took a little time to reflect while we were up there (there is a chapter coming on this very "ingredient".) You can't help but do this while you sit on top of the world with the view in front of you. You are reminded about how small you really are and the powerful forces that exist on this planet that could only be in place due to God. And since I was up there, I took the time to have a brief discussion with Him, thinking that it would be that much easier for Him to hear me since I was closer to Him way up there in the mountains. We soaked up as much as we could and decided to head back down on the train to visit the town and have some refreshments. Sitting at the sidewalk cafés sipping coffee or a wine (depending on the time of day) soaking in the environment and people watching is one of my favorite and most relaxing activities.

Once back in town, the kids played around a while on the

old train while Jules and her friend (who made the trip with us) did a little looking around in the shops. Since it was about 7:30 in the evening at this point we had to make a decision, do we head back to Coppet for dinner or sit in the cafes and have a light snack? The cafés were just too tempting and won out. We bought the kids an ice cream cone and settled in at a little café. Julie and had a "café" (coffee) while Jenn ordered up a half bottle of regional Pinot Noir. To tide our hungry bellies, we also ordered a Fondu d' Fromage (Cheese Fondu). It was huge and we could not stop eating it. "I'd just like to say that Fondu is delicious. It fills you up on a nice alpine evening" (a rip off of one of my favorite lines of Ricky Bobby from the Movie "Talladega Nights".) I can't wait to try Fondu d' Chocolat.

Well that about sums up yesterday's events. I have just finished my cup of Nescafe and need to head upstairs to get ready for today's events. I believe we are going to take a

Before moving on to the next "ingredient," I think it is important to note that not all experiences must be as grand and as elaborate as the one mentioned above that we were so fortunate to share. Many people don't have such options. Experiences are all about you and your loved one and what you consider an experience. You or your loved one may also not be in the best physical condition due to the treatment and/or the Cancer itself. Going on trips, hikes, even local outings may be out of the question. Playing a board game or cards at home with the family could be a cherished family experience. Starting a tradition of movie night (or day depending on when you are feeling your best), holding each other in bed, reading a book to each other that you both enjoy, or even just sitting outside on a porch swing holding hands while you enjoy a beautiful day and a light breeze could be a grand experience that each of you will enjoy and remember forever, regardless of the outcome of the medical aspect and outcome of the Cancer treatments.

Remember where I stated earlier that we are all going to pass at some point. No one gets out alive. All Cancer does is give you an idea of a potential timeframe of when that MIGHT happen. Cancer's goal, if I can give it a personality, is to terrorize you and "steal your joy". It wants you to live in depression, fear, anxiety and sadness. If you do not let this happen, YOU steal Cancer's joy. How awesome is that?!

Chapter 6

Ingredient: Multiple Tablespoons of Reflection

Looking back on this time of my life this is an "ingredient" that I wish I had paid more attention to and maybe even added several more Tablespoons to the mixing vat. I was so busy with caring for Julie and spending time with the kids, I never spent much thought appreciating the time.

There were several times that I started to keep a journal. Julie and I had an idea that we would take a half hour each night and write our thoughts about the day in those journals. They would be personal journals where we could document to ourselves our most intimate feelings, thoughts, fears, hopes, joys, etc. and capture all of that for reflection in the future. I agreed that it would be a great idea and the next day we went off to a popular bookstore to look for fancy journal books that we would use to chronicle the thoughts referenced above each day. We did a great job of this for about 3-4 weeks. I actually think Julie did a better job than I did and kept it up for a few more weeks. Looking back this is one of my biggest regrets, as I later learned how important it is to live in the moment and appreciate and take in all that is presented to you throughout each waking moment. The good and the bad.

After Julie WON her battle with Cancer, I found myself struggling with life and being "normal" again. What is "normal" anyway? I once had a

friend tell me, "Don't worry about normal. It is nothing more than a setting on the dryer."
Along the way, I met a great man, a Zen Guru of sorts, named Wayne. You probably have noted from previous chapters that I was raised and am of the Christian faith (more on this later). I don't believe that Wayne is Christian, but can't say for sure as we never talked about that directly, but I do know that he believes in a higher authority of some sort and is the kindest and most peaceful spirit anyone could ever meet. In one casual encounter I was approaching him, and we were just about to exchange a passing greeting and he stopped in his tracks and said to me, "One moment." He turned to look at a plant growing along the sidewalk that had the most amazing flower with very vibrant colors emanating from its petals. Wayne stopped and leaned in for a closer look and took in the moment. He then turned to me and said, "Isn't it beautiful? It is just growing here for all of us to see and is an amazing creation of the world." He then greeted and we shared a brief conversation, but I could not stop thinking about how observant he was to the "moment" and taking in his surroundings AND pausing long enough to enjoy it, even just for a moment.

A year or so later, through the power of social media, I learned that Wayne was in Alaska hiking off the grid and taking in all the "moments" he could in what I certainly believe is the last earthly frontier. As luck would have it, I was in Alaska at the same time for business reasons. I reached out to Wayne and let him know I was there, and would he be near Anchorage anytime that week. He quickly replied that he would be, and we should meet up. We agreed that we would meet up in the evening when I finished work (at this time it was mid-summer and the sun never really sets there during that time of year) and we would go on a local hike to an area called "Flat Top Mountain."

Flat Top mountain is exactly what it sounds like. It is part of the mountain range that borders the southern part of the city and it's very distinct in its appearance. As all the mountains around it have peaks this one looks like it's peak has been sawed off. It is a hike of moderate exertion and takes an hour to an hour and half to ascend from the trail head. Once you crest the "summit," if there is one on a flat-topped mountain, you are treated to wonderous views of Anchorage and the Cook Inlet body of water. On this evening there was a subtle breeze and the day was crystal clear. You could even see both peaks of Mount Denali in the distance that was hundreds of miles away in one direction, and Mount Redoubt (an active volcano) in the other direction. We talked the whole way up stopping a few times for me to catch my breath (he was in much better hiking shape than me at the time) and for him to stop and take a few pictures of local wildflowers that once again I would have walked right by. When we reached the top, we both went silent. We sat a few feet apart from each other and said nothing. We took in the views and spent at least an hour in silent thought and reflection. We looked at the water, listened to birds, watched the "crazies" launch themselves off the top of the mountain with parasails and glide around on the updrafts. We were in the moment meditating, and not letting the stresses of the world absorb and dominate our lives. When we were done, I felt lighter and so refreshed.

I wish I had done more of this when the battle with Cancer was won. It truly would have been a punch in the groin to Cancer. It is sad that as I look back through the blog, looking for a post that truly represents time in personal reflection, I struggled to find one. The closest one I found was a tribute I wrote to Julie on Mother's Day of 2007. Please read below.

Happy Mother's Day Julie - Sunday, May 13, 2007

My Dearest Julie,

Happy Mother's Day to a beautiful lady and mother to three of the luckiest children on earth.

It amazes me to watch you in your role as a mom. How you manage to put them first in everything you do. How you successfully divert their attention when they are starting to fight with each other, how you come up with all the arts and crafts (or as Hallie used to call them arts and crabs) for them to do on rainy days, and how you spend hours toting them around to birthdays and making sure they get to stay for cake and the Spanish speaking clown, even though you are dog tired. The list goes on and on.

You do the little things for the kids that a dad would never think of, like putting little messages on the napkins in their lunch boxes so that they know that they are loved and special. I sit back in amazement of your passion for being a mother wishing I could be half the parent you are. You don't even need to tell the kids that you love them, because you exude that love for them in your actions and in your eyes.

Kendall and Jackson are still too young to truly appreciate how fantastic their mother really is, but I know they have a pretty good idea. Hallie on the other hand is starting to truly understand her fortune in having you as a mother. The times spent with her at the Daisy Scout meetings and *outings, working in the garden with you, and the patience you have in combing out her hair after the shower... she definitely prefers you to do that vs. mean old dad who just yanks that brush through her hair.*

I think Hallie has already probably done a pretty good job of showing her gratitude by fixing you breakfast in bed (read: toast) and I am sure that Jack has followed her lead and has done an adequate job in recognizing you today. However, on behalf of Kendall and myself

THANK YOU FOR BEING THE FANTASTIC MOTHER THAT YOU ARE TO THIS FAMILY.

I am sorry that I missed this weekend with you and am in fact writing this on the airplane home. I can't wait to get home and wrap my arms around you, Julie. I LOVE YOU.

PS ... Happy Mother's Day to you too, Mom. Thank you for always being there for me, to celebrate the good times with me and help support me through the tough ones. I can never repay you for being the person that you have been to me for the last 11 plus years. Thank you from the bottom of my heart.

Chapter 7

Ingredient: Add a liberal amount of Treats

Similar to Humor where I said in the early stages, I felt like there should be no humor and then when I realized humor was not just OK, but needed, I still felt guilty for a long time in laughing at anything I found funny or cracking a joke. "Treats" are a similar concept. Treat yourself periodically to things you truly enjoy doing. In some ways, they are very similar to the "experiences" I discussed earlier but there is a subtle distinction. Experiences are more or less planned and sometimes become regular traditions or even routines. "Treats," on the other hand, tend to be spontaneous and very much unplanned events or activities that you truly enjoy doing.

For example, I remember on, spring evening the weather forecast for the weekend was supposed to be spectacular. We were in the middle of our two-week Spring period in Houston that has very "California Like" weather. Julie said to me, "Why don't you use tomorrow and treat yourself to a round of golf with your dad or a couple of your friends? You have not played since before the diagnosis." My response was to let the Cancer terrorist rule my initial response. No babe, I want to spend the time with you because in the back of my mind I had that thought of how many days do I have left with her and I don't want to waste one. Again, no one knows how many days we have left on this Earth. As hard as it is to face reality, anyone reading this book could have many years left to live but equally true is that this very day could be your last day. From a human error standpoint, accidents claim lives every day. But even more sobering to me is that very few people know what their medical prognosis is for heart disease, stroke or brain aneurism. No one says, "I have only a 54 percent chance of surviving a heart attack later this year." The real truth is that all Cancer does is put the fear of a real timeline of your (or your loved one's) mortality in your head and dominate your thoughts. This domination then paralyzes your action. I play golf usually once a week these days and don't think twice about "treating myself to a round" at this point because I still don't know how much time I have left with anyone that is important to me in my life (e.g. family and friends) that matter.

I then tried the option of declining her suggestion by insisting I could not burden her with watching all three kids. Her response was simply, "They are my kids. They are no burden. Besides, it will give me some time with them to just do mommy things with them and have a special time with them." So, without any other excuses to pull out from my sleeve, I reluctantly called the local course asked if they had any tee times, which they did, and secured a late morning start. I then called my dad and a couple buddies and twisted their arms (sarcasm) into joining me. It was a great day and I had forgotten how much I enjoyed the "guy time" of congratulating each other on the rare great shot and laughing our butts off at the more common bad shot. Then we spent a couple hours at the "19th hole" where we all got a birdie, so to speak, by enjoying a couple cold brewskis (obligatory post round activity) and rehashing every shot of every hole.

> Side bar … Most women find it amazing that men who golf can remember every shot of every hole, how good or bad the shot was, what the situation was and the end result of not only their round but the other 3 members in their foursome - but can never remember to fix the leaky faucet their wife has asked them to do 77 times over a three month period. However, as men, I will say that we find it equally interesting that women can remember where, and when, they bought every item of clothing, or pair of shoes, and how much it cost including tax … AND every item of clothing they ever bought was on sale, so they saved a ton of money. Are there any women's clothing items in stores ever that are full price? I don't think so.

> *See, humor is truly important to me! But, I digress … back to liberal amounts of "Treats."*

Very similar to the earlier chapter, where I peeled myself off of the couch and helped Jules paint the room, for a brief moment in time, Cancer did not dominate my thoughts when I was with my dad and the boys on the golf course. Cancer had nothing to do with it. It was about TREATING MYSLEF to something that was fun with family and friends.

Julie took to treating herself to various items as well. The occasional girls' night out where she would go to foodie style restaurants with her lifelong girlfriends and do that girl talk thing that I am completely and supremely unqualified to discuss. I suspect they talked about how great of a husband I was, bra fitting, and "The Bachelorette" … but I am just speculating. Other times, maybe she would treat herself to a trip to the hair salon even though her hair was thinning and there was not much she could do with it. Still a treat. Another treat she would enjoy was walking around the lake in our neighborhood and getting some exercise while having some good alone time.

Treats are how you and your loved ones define them. A spur of the moment trip to the local ice cream shop and loading up on mix-ins count as a treat. A quiet time on the porch swing with your favorite musician playing on your Bluetooth speaker with a light breeze blowing is a treat. Watching a movie on Netflix or binge watching a great show is a treat. Going for a run, the gym, or a yoga class are all treats to yourself. Treats are what you make them. That's the beauty of them, no one can define them but you. Once again you are in control and Cancer is in the basement pouting because it is not dominating your thoughts and activities. Good! Pout away Cancer because no one cares how you feel.

The following blog post is something that I treated myself to with Julie's blessing, of course. I have since retired from the advocation of basketball officiating but at the time it truly was a passion for me and a treat every time I took the floor (I might have some former coaches I worked for and thousands of fans who might not agree) but similar to Cancer's feelings, their feelings didn't register with me.

It's that Time of Year Again – Sunday, November 5, 2006

Well November has arrived and is normally a very exciting time of year for me as it marks the beginning of basketball season. Those that know me, know that I am a Collegiate (Small College) and High School basketball referee and I am very passionate about it. I started officiating basketball eight years ago as a way to get re-acquainted with a sport that was so much a part of my life growing up. I played competitively all the way through my sophomore year in college. My playing career ended when I suffered a torn knee ligament toward the end of a game.

I decided that I still wanted to be a part of the game and officiating was the only option that meshed with my profession as I did not have the time to coach. I fell in love with officiating from the moment I stepped onto the floor with the whistle and the stripes and it has been a very important part of our lives ever since. I enjoy the camaraderie (many of my closest friends these days are those that I have met through officiating), the mental challenge it provides me, the physical exercise and the sense of giving back to the game I love. Julie enjoys the game fees that show up in the mailbox throughout the season.

However, this year is different. I am not nearly as excited about this season, and I imagine you can venture a guess as to why. In fact, I gave very serious consideration to taking the year off to focus on my family and Julie during this time, as officiating is a huge time commitment. However, at the insistence of Julie and with the encouragement of my family, they convinced me that

I should continue on with officiating this year as I normally would have.

In a post I made earlier [I will come back to this post later], I spoke of Jimmy Valvano and his battle with Cancer. I stated that even though he had Cancerous lesions all over his body, he refused to let Cancer define and control his life. Had I taken the season completely off, I would have LET Cancer do just that to us. Truth is, I need officiating as a "treat to myself" and as an outlet and an opportunity to think about something I truly enjoy for a couple hours, a couple days per week. It is more or less a break from Cancer for me and something to help keep me physically and mentally healthy. So, with that thought in mind, I took my college and high school schedules, discussed what kind of help we may need with Julie and the kids with our families and I prepared for the season.

My first game was this past Thursday night. It was a junior college game at Lamar State which is only seventy miles away in Port Arthur, TX (I say only because, it is nothing for us to drive three and half hours each way for one of these college games). It was especially tough to leave for this game with Julie being in the hospital, however, I was assigned to work this game with one of my good referee friends, so we rode to the game together. It is a good thing we did, because our third partner was supposed to meet us there and he never showed (We work all games with three referees, so the fact that we had to work one with only two is noteworthy!)

Anyway, I got through the game (it was an easy one as the home team completely blew the visiting team out of the gym), I was able to focus on something else for three or four hours, earned some extra cash and I was able to get back up to the hospital to be with Julie by 10:30 p.m. ... just before she fell asleep.

Julie has always been very supportive of my officiating "hobby" as she knows the enjoyment and satisfaction I get from it. Thank you, Julie, (and family) for convincing me to treat myself to this hobby and continue on this year as it is a great outlet for me. As of right now, it is the right decision.

Love to All,

-Brendan

Chapter 8

Ingredient: Drip in Tears as Needed

I spent a lot of time earlier and throughout this book talking about the value of humor. I have also tried to inject a little bit of my humor throughout several chapters since. But for now, I would like to focus on dealing and/or coping with your grief and fear that is associated with such a diagnosis.

The body, and more specifically for this discussion, the brain, is wonderfully geared to cleanse the body of problems that plague us and the emotions that bring you to the point in which tears flow is but one of those functions. Fear, grief, and physical pain are all conditions that life throws at us that might invoke us to cry "real tears."

When these emotions hit you, it is important to let the body do what it is supposed to do. Given our cultural mores, personal observation, and my own experience this is much harder for men than it is for women. Men are taught at an early age to suck it up, be a man and never show any signs of being vulnerable. To let people see this is perceived as a sign of weakness. Women, on the other hand, have a slight advantage in our culture of being freer to publicly show emotion. It is actually accepted and excepted for a woman to show fear and sadness and be vulnerable. It is part of being feminine and when they are having these feelings are told "It's ok, let it out." Therefore, it is my belief that women are at a distinct advantage when dealing with these situations and staying emotionally healthy. If men cry where others can see them, they feel embarrassed which actually compounds the negative effects of the emotions one is feeling because you start to feel "not strong enough,", "you are showing that you are a weak man," and an overall failure in managing your emotions. The ironic thing is by not allowing yourself to grieve and let others know you are hurting and scared is the very definition of not managing your emotions.

Now you may be a little bit confused because at the beginning of this book, I talked about how I cried and cried upon hearing her diagnosis. And how I cried most of the next day while she was on a mission to paint my son's room. But understand this was only within the safety of the company of my wife. That evening, when I went to the hospital, I sucked it up and put some drops in my eyes to try and reduce the swelling for when we got to the hospital and we were in the company of strangers. I could not "afford" to let strangers in the form of other patients or medical staff see me being weak. When we returned home that night, my family was there and there was absolutely no crying. I did not eat as I had no appetite and I was clearly not myself, but no way was I going to let my parents see one tear flow from my eyes. I was the man of the house and I was in control - except that I wasn't. Why I could not afford to do this is strictly a function of our cultural values and the synthetic need to try and hide my feelings and emotions.

Now here is the proof that this was a huge issue for me. I have read through the whole blog and there is not one post where I mention I broke down in tears. There are a couple references to them from Julie which I will capture below. But I will follow that up with a couple stories that I remember like yesterday where I just flat broke down.

> *Acceptance - Thursday, January 11, 2007 (authored by Julie)*
>
> *Wow, What a week. As you know, Monday was rough. I can't lie. Hearing that even though we had taken the most aggressive chemotherapy treatment available for Melanoma and it didn't work... wow ... it was hard. It put me in an emotional vacuum that day. Everything just got sucked out of me. I felt as though I was back at my original diagnosis. Here we were, all ready for the hospital stay, which takes a lot of emotional preparedness as well as logistical (with the lives of three kids to keep as normal as possible), and we were basically told to take our*

*luggage home and go consider
our options. I am sure my post
from Monday night rambled ...
it was hard thinking straight.*

*Tuesday was also a rough one.
All those emotions that had
been sucked out the day before
came flooding back once I had
time to think about it.
Thoughts of my own mortality,
and, "what is wrong with MY
body that it didn't respond,"
worrying about the kids and
praying I am there for them for
as long as possible. I didn't feel
like talking to anyone, and if I
did, I would probably start
crying. Poor Gerald (note:
another Melanoma patient we
had befriended at MDACC), I
called him at the hospital and
the flood gates just opened ...
hopefully he was still in the
throes of Chemo Brain and
won't remember it! Even
Brendan noticed it and kept
telling me, "you gotta keep
fighting it," and, "hang on." If
we hadn't already had a
backup plan in place, I would
probably STILL be curled up in
a ball crying and feeling
sorrow for our family.*

Luckily, by Wednesday I was getting better. I was facing forward, not dwelling on the mishaps. As Brendan put It, maybe the MDACC stone in the path was to keep everything in check. Keep the Melanoma under control until we found the next stone. I mean, we are lucky that the disease hasn't progressed. WE are still working with the same tumors we had before. NO other areas are affected, my lymph nodes are still clean, and my brain is clean ... Praise God!

I cannot stress the importance of having a plan to fall back on. When I first, started this, before I even started the clinical trial, I spoke with a woman who beat Melanoma ten years ago (through a vaccine) and one of the things she told me was that the way she has kept it at bay for so long was to always stay one step ahead. I guess I didn't fully understand what she was telling me at the time, but I do now.

Yesterday, B and I had to go up to the hospital to pick up paperwork from the skin center to take to the Mary Crowley Center in Dallas, and I got into a conversation with a woman (as I tend to do, got that trait from my Dad!). We talked a little bit and I asked her who she was here with. She said her brother in-law had recently been diagnosed and was about to start a clinical trial. From what she was telling me I think it will be the same clinical trial I did the first time with the addition of one drug because he has brain tumors. I told her about our history and the Oncavex trial we are about to start. Kendall started crying and I stepped away to go feed her. As Brendan and I started to leave she and her husband came over to ask how we had found out about the clinical trial we are about to start ... Well, that got us going! We gave them the same advice Karen Velasquez gave me so many months ago ... stay ahead of it. Have a backup plan ready, go to the National Institutes of Health web site, find out what is out there, how well it is working and what you can do to be a part of the program.

Even though we were praying (and assuming) that bio chemo would work, Plan C was waiting in the wings. If Plan C doesn't work, we will be ready to move ahead with MDX-010. I like my sister Sherri's "recipe" analogy. There are thousands of recipes for lasagna ... we just have to find the right one for our family.

I would be remiss if I didn't also point out that we had my father-in-law to help. Dan is an engineer, and all the standard engineer-isms apply, save for a pocket protector ... and I don't think he breaks out the slide rule NEARLY as often as he used to! Every meeting he attended with us he dutifully took out his note cards and started writing. He wrote down every drug name, every hospital referral, asked questions and then went back home and did research. Brendan and I started out trying to do this ourselves, but when you are sitting in that small clinic room listening to the enormity of what is being said to you it is hard to even fathom taking notes. He got us

*set up at the Crowley Center
and even though I didn't want
to pursue it until AFTER we
knew what the bio was doing
… I didn't want to have
negative "it's not working"
thoughts … we went in my last
off week. So glad we did. Even
on Monday's trip home from
the hospital Brendan was
already making phone calls to
find out what we need to do to
start the Oncavex.*

*All that being said, I am back
to my normal self. There are
moments of, "Aw Geez, this
really sucks!" Hey, I am not a
Stepford Wife … sometimes I
get scared! But don't think I
am not ready to keep on
fighting and finding just the
right lasagna. Cancer doesn't
stand a chance!!*

Love to all and God Bless

YAY GOD!!!

Julie

**NOTE - I realize not everything in the above
post deals with tears and grief. But I have
decided to include all posts in their entirety
because you can see that many of the**

ingredients that I have listed can be found in splashes throughout. Additionally, I find that some of the other topics discussed within maybe helpful to those who currently find themselves in the situation that we were in in 2006 and 2007.

Now as far as my story and dealing with my emotions. As I stated in the beginning, I felt unsafe in doing so. Except for the moments after diagnosis and a few times in between, I held it all in. The pressure of the grief building inside me was akin to a volcano. If you do not relieve the pressure, little by little the grief, fear and anxiety will explode with enormous magnitude.

But before I give you my story in terms of adding drips of tears as necessary, I need to provide context and introduce you to Jessie as she is integral to the story.

The People You Meet …-
Thursday March 01, 2007

One of the "good "things that have come out of our encounter with the big "C" is the people we have met on the "road" whom we would have not met otherwise. Rachel and Gerald Boudreaux, Marilyn and Jim Ryan and a host of others. However, I have been long overdue to introduce the "Army" to Miss Jessie.

Jessie was our nurse practitioner during our many recent in-patient stays at MDACC. We quickly forged a bond and friendship with Jessie, and she was truly a bright spot in the darkness that chemo treatments and in-patient stays create. In fact, we lucked into having her as our NP during our first emergency admission while on the Lenalidomide trial because she was on duty. She was not supposed to be our regular NP based on our doctor. However, after our first stay, she petitioned to stay on as our NP for every other subsequent stay because we got along so well. And, if she had not petitioned, we surely would have requested her!

Working in personnel, I have a pretty good read on people and their job satisfaction. I could tell right away that Jessie truly loves her job and gets a lot of satisfaction out of helping people manage through very difficult days. She always had words of

Now that you have met Jessie, we can get on with my addition of healthy tears to the mixing vat. We were several months into treatment; we got another round of disappointing test results and Julie was admitted to the hospital. Jessie seemed "off"
 that day and is the reason I wanted to introduce you to her before I went into this story. When she left the room, I looked at Julie and asked her if she thought Jessie was different. Maybe she was having a bad day, but Jessie never let that show even if she was. Julie

agreed that she was different in mood, so I left the room to go seek her out. She was at the nurse's station and I asked if she was OK. She just kind of looked at me for a moment but I could see it in her eyes that things were not. She asked me to come around the counter and she showed me the latest scans that Julie had gone through. Not only were they not good, but the tumors were growing. A positive prognosis was eroding, and I could see her emotions welling up. I stayed stoic and outwardly strong and went back into the room. But Julie knew better, she said, "the news is REALLY not good is it … Be honest with me." So I broke down and cried. She on the other hand did not. More to come on that later. Once I pulled myself together again, I excused myself under some pretense of needing to go get something to eat or check on something for work, I don't recall. I just knew I had to leave.

I went to a quiet break room, that surprisingly, no one was occupying. I reached into my pocket and pulled out my medical benefits card and my phone and I stared at them for what seemed like hours. On the back of the card was the Employee Assistance Program number. I dialed halfway through the number several times and cancelling the call as I knew I needed help but could not commit myself to getting it. In my head that meant I was mentally weak. Finally, I dialed all the digits of the 800 number and let it ring. I went through the phone tree options to get to the mental health help and counselors. When I finally got the live person on the phone, she answered politely with her name and asked how she could be of assistance. I just remember bursting into tears and slobbering the words, "I just can't do it by myself anymore. I NEED help. Please help me." It sounds ridiculous, but I can't tell you how cathartic just that very moment was. Obviously that one moment didn't solve my immediate problem but I had crossed the bridge of knowing I needed help and went so far as asking for it. And here is the greatest part, I felt no less of a man after having done so.

The EAP employee stayed on the phone with me and asked me what was going on. I explained my situation to her and said that I have been trying to cope for several months and tough it out. We talked for 30 to 45 minutes, I don't remember and when it was all done, she reassured me that I had made a big step and more importantly, the right step. She assisted me in getting an appointment in the next couple of days and we disconnected the phone.

I pulled myself back together (or at least I thought I had) and went back to Julie's room. She smiled at me because she could sense something different in me from when I had left. She said, "where did you really go?" She could always tell when I was not being truthful! I told her I finally broke down and called for help. I had an appointment with a psychologist in a couple days. She smiled and told me to come to her bed. She reached up, put her arms around me, hugged me and whispered in my ear, "I am so happy and proud that you did that. I have been hoping and praying you would get some help in coping for a long time. But I know you and knew that if you were going to do it, it had to be your idea and on your terms."

Now remember, this ingredient is difficult and like in many recipes, some spices are very strong and too much can ruin a very good recipe even if you get everything else right. Ever have a dish that was way too salty? A bowl of chili with too much cumin? It tastes bad right? But it also doesn't taste good if you don't add any at all! It is delicate and the "Tears" are the critical spice in this dish. You can put too much in and Cancer is always in your ear screaming, "MORE TEARS! MORE TEARS! YOU DEFINITELY DON'T HAVE ENOUGH TEARS!" Cancer is the terrorist and wants to ruin your recipe and cause you to lose. But don't add enough, and the body starts to work against itself. Therefore, you must work a very careful balance. Add them when necessary but do not allow yourself to get a heavy hand and add tears to the dish whenever Cancer yells, "MORE TEARS DAMN IT!" A drip here and a drip there is healthy and all you need. Remember, your recipe is almost complete, and Cancer is losing. Don't open the door and give it hope that it can make a comeback and actually have a chance at winning this thing after all.

Chapter 9

Ingredient: Fold in plenty of Documentation

People have often said, if you or a loved one ever have Cancer, don't waste it. This is difficult to understand until you have lived it and then the advice becomes crystal clear. Having the diagnosis forces you to live every moment; you want to be able to look back afterward and say that you did just that. You will always have the memories in your head but unfortunately, they fade or distort over time. A supervisor of mine once said, "A short pencil is far better than a long memory," and 12 years later I can say he is right. This book would be almost impossible for me to write if not for the book that was printed off our electronic blog before it was removed by the host. For that I am grateful.

Reading through this blog on a periodic basis reminds me of times I have forgotten, at worst case, and in the best case, fills in gaps of the memories that I do have. I see pictures of the kids interacting with both of us at such precious and tender ages. It brings back raw emotions both good and bad, but I would argue (and will demonstrate later) that regardless of the type of emotion that the entry evokes it is good. Bad emotions are as needed as the good emotions, as they are part of the human experience, and over time, define who we are as a person. Events that trigger the hard emotions, I would argue, help shape us to be more empathetic and caring individuals who are better at understanding others and encourages you to be more giving of yourself. To put it more bluntly, they help check your ego. It is easier to explain why the good emotions are important to relive. When you find yourself reading and realize that you are unconsciously smiling at a memory, the dopamine released in your brain immediately puts you into a very natural high that will reinvigorate you for the rest of the day or even week.

Documentation, however, is not just blogs. One thing I personally regret is not taking more photos during that time period and even more specifically videos. Now keep in mind, cell phone technology then was not as it is today. Almost all of us have a camera AND video recorder in our pants pocket or purse. Additionally, today we have almost unlimited storage capacity with cloud storage that just hovers around us in an invisible medium that we can recall whenever we wish for our viewing. When we were having our experience with Cancer, I had a small Sony Cybershot camera that I would carry around with me and take the occasional video or photo with and then later have the extra step of downloading them to the computer. The problem was that we were so busy with the kids, treatments, doctor appointments and life, that many times I would forget to download them. Sometimes I did, and I have those, other times, things got inadvertently recorded over. Sometimes I wanted to capture something and didn't have enough space … and worst of all, I am guilty of losing a memory card or two along the way.

Today's technology solves all of that for almost everyone and you can capture as much as you need. But here is my caution to each and every one reading this book - don't capture everything on photo and/or video. Don't live this part of your life witnessing it through a camera lens. There is a fine line to walk as to how much to capture. While you are capturing moments don't forget to experience them.

I was recently watching a golf tournament and Tiger Woods was on the tee box getting ready tee off. Almost everyone knows that Tiger is a world-renowned celebrity and athlete and arguably the best to ever play the game. He revolutionized many aspects of the game and for years people were in awe of how far he could drive the ball off the tee. He will be in the Golf Hall of Fame and will go down as a legend of the game. As he stood on the tee box, I noticed the gallery surrounding him was 20-30 people deep equating to hundreds of people surrounding him. Almost every single person was holding their phone up above their head trying to video the shot. I kept thinking to myself take a picture if you want to remember you were there next to him, or a quick 15-second video clip, but then put the phone away and savor the moment and watch the man hit the ball through the lens of your eye versus the lens of a phone camera. You can Google or YouTube him hitting the ball on video anytime you want. You can rarely go back and watch him hit a ball in person and fully appreciate you are watching a legend play the game live right in front of you.

The same is true for picture and video of your life with your family while you are fighting back against Cancer. Take enough video and pictures to evoke the emotions and fill in the gaps for your memories, but then let your brain take over and remember the experience that you took in while in the moment.

Journals are fabulous tools as well to look back on and I truly wish I as well as Julie had taken this medium more seriously and applied much more effort into it. Our blog was primarily designed to capture significant events, treatments, and overall progress against the disease. What journals do a better job of, is capturing raw thoughts, emotions and musings. Better yet it is in your own handwriting. There is a certain intimacy created with those memories using this medium. Keeping a journal takes commitment and discipline. Time each day needs to be committed to spending time in thought and chronicling those thoughts accordingly. Julie and I tried this as I have mentioned earlier and the time of day we carved out was when we crawled into bed. We thought this would be a great idea as we would have the full day to gather our thoughts. However, it was a bad idea in that we were generally exhausted by the time we climbed in and pulled the covers over us. The last thing we wanted to do was pen a page or two of our deepest thoughts and feelings. We were successful for a couple of weeks but it slowly waned until we did no more ... actually, I found out later that Julie did a slightly better job than I did much later.

If you choose to keep a journal, pick a time that you can carve out, roughly around the same time each day, and stick with it. Science shows that it takes roughly 28-30 days for habits to form. This coincidentally is why many people fail at diet and exercise programs. They get going and after a week or two see a pound or two drop but don't feel like they have gained enough ground on their goal, wondering why it is not being shed quicker. They then throw their hands in the air and give up. If you start a journal, make a concerted effort to keep it up for a month. Trust that once the habit develops it will stick and you will have this journal to look back on for years to come. Another opportunity to "not waste your Cancer."

Halloween 2007 - Friday, November 02, 2007

I am not going to start this post about Cancer .... I will save that for later. Instead, lets address the fun that is associated with Halloween which is made even more special in the fact that Hallie (yes, that is where she got her name) was born on this day 7 years ago.

The kids decided to dress as follows:

Hallie - Witch (I am not sure if she was a good one or not)

Jackson - Black Spiderman with muscles (No, he has not even seen the movie)

Kendall - A Lioness (All of our kids have worn this costume for their first Halloween)

Sidney (our dog) = Red/ Blue Spiderman (Bwahahahahaha)

Yes, Kendall has thrown herself on the floor in a crying fit and wouldn't wear the lion "hat" but as soon as we hit the street and put the pumpkin bucket in her hand... she was ready to go!

We have a great neighborhood for trick or treating in that it is gated, which keeps traffic to a minimum and most of the "riff raff" (read trouble making teenagers) out. And many of the neighbors really get into it with elaborate decorations and even a 3-D haunted house constructed in a garage!

Hallie's birthday celebration started on Saturday where she held a "Harry Potter" themed birthday. Many thanks to Nana for making all the capes for the event and to Ebony the Super-Nanny, for volunteering to come over on her day off and help! The kids had a blast running around in the backyard and playing while the adults sat out on our new screened in porch. (Many thanks to team DPC for that.)

Sunday evening, we all dressed up into our costumes and headed over to St. Jerome's Pumpkin Fest. It is a Halloween party complete with a big kids haunted house (which was awesome ... good job 8th graders) and little kids haunted house so that the little tykes wouldn't feel left out! Julie motored around in her wheelchair with her witch's hat, I got all camo'ed up and went as a hunter (no gun ... I am one bad dude as I told Jack. I take down game with my bare hands!) and of course the kids put on their costumes (except for Kendall, but she had a blast without it anyway).

The birthday continued on through last night with friends, my grandmother (who is currently in town), and of course my folks. Hallie mopped up on birthday goodies, cake, and plenty of candy.

I am working on uploading all of the pictures to our Flickr account and will post the link here shortly once that is accomplished. However, I am getting all kinds of error messages at the moment. I actually think it is a problem with the internet connection here at MDACC ...

NOTE - The rest of this post deals with her latest Cancer update so I will omit.

Again, I know I said I was going to try and limit the blog post entries to one per chapter as support for the points I am trying to make in the chapter. However, in this chapter we are talking about the ingredient Documentation so why not add just a bit more documentation in the chapter. Below is an entry that Julie penned wishing her youngest baby girl a very Happy Birthday….

Happy Birthday Baby! - Sunday, July 22, 2007

Happy Birthday Kendall! You turned one on June 19th and even though this post is on July 21st, Mommy wanted to wish you a Happy Day … Sorry for the delay, but you are the third. You should be glad we got around to doing this at all! Now, if I can only get that baby book of yours up to date before you graduate from high school! Someday you and Aunt Sherri can trade, "I was the last" woes. I am sure it will make for some good therapy sessions!

We had your one-year checkup this past week. Four shots and a TB test ... which you HATED! Your stats were 18 pounds and (I think) 24 inches long. You rank in the tenth percentile for weight. Thirtieth for height and fortieth for head size. Not quite proportionate, but I am sure with time that will even out! To me you are perfect!

Your personality is fun and easy going. You aren't scared to get right in the thick of whatever Hallie and Jack are doing and even though you and Sidney see eye to eye you just push her out of the way if she tries to get too pushy with you. You have no fear. You love being silly. When you think you are being funny you crinkle your nose and squint your eyes.

You have a great way of communicating what you want. My favorite is your request to go outside (which you do A LOT). You find your shoes (the cheap purple and pink Wal-Mart shoes are your favorite.) You bring them to whatever grownup is handy. Give them to said grown up, plop your padded bottom on the ground and grunt a little. We all know exactly what you want! The other day you wanted so badly to go outside, and it was POURING DOWN rain. I thought, well, let's go to the door and I will SHOW you that now is not a good time. We stood there looking at *the rain then you looked up at me and pointed your shoes in my direction. I don't think you got it.*

You started walking at 10 months. ON THE DAY of being 10 months! We beat cousin Addie and that was our goal, really. Looks like all that time in the Excer-Saucer paid off!

We happened to be picking up Jack at school and I sat you on the floor in his classroom. You moved to a squatting position, then stood up ... took a few steps ... a few more, then squatted back down again. Within a few weeks you were running.

Oh, and your climbing abilities ... I would be remiss if I didn't mention those. I call you Monkey Girl. I think you have fingers on your feet! Climbing on the couches and chairs is a breeze. In addition, you have climbed on top of the kitchen table AND out of your crib. The crib thing isn't a fluke either. You have done that numerous times. The first time it happened I had put you down for a nap and you fussed and fussed. I didn't think much of it because you USUALLY pitch a fit when it is time for a nap. This time, however, Hallie came down and asked me, "Is Kendall supposed to be on the floor, because I peeked in on her and she is sitting on the floor." "No, Hal … she is SUPPOSED to be in the crib."

Kendall, know that Mommy loves you. Your first year has been amazing and you have brightened our lives immensely. In your little life I already see in you an appreciation of humor, an outdoor spirit and LOTS of gumption. I look forward to seeing the woman you become.

All my love (well, I will share some with Hallie, Jack and Daddy but you get a Lyons share!)

-Mommy

I have shared these posts with you to show that documentation during your battle with Cancer should not always be about Cancer. Focus on ALL of the good things in your life and ignore the Cancer for extended periods of time. Notice what your kids are doing and watch in awe as they develop and grow. Pay attention to the world. Remember, earlier, my friend and his amazing ability to live in the moment and let the natural beauty of the world fill his spirit and soul? Whether it be a small flower, a bird singing in the morning, people watching or taking in the magic of the diversity in all of us. Do not fixate on Cancer, for if you do, guess who is winning?

Chapter 10

Ingredient: Heaping helpings of Faith

You may have noticed that many of the blog postings are ended with the phrase "YAY GOD." You have probably ascertained at this point that we are people of faith, and more specifically, the Christian faith.

However, I want to be clear that I am not proselytizing. Many different people worship in their own way as there are many religions out there. From the more traditional, Christian, Jewish, Hindu and Muslim to the more untraditional that are far too many to even begin to pen a list. I go back to my friend Wayne, whom I mentioned earlier, that I went hiking with in Alaska. I would not describe him as a man of traditional religion based on what I have seen and observed (again, I have never asked) but I would describe him as a very spiritual man. He does believe in some higher power, some larger force that is moving us through this thing called life and the entire cosmos … Wayne, if you are reading this, "Namaste."

I have to believe that there is something more than just the very few years we have on this earth. It matters not if you live 8 years or 105 years. In the grand scheme of things, it is a very short time period regardless of the number of years you actually do live. I don't profess to know what is next. I have my beliefs based on my religion and I think everyone should have their beliefs based on however they choose to think about what comes next. I believe there is something more than this very short existence of being a kid, spending 40 years working, growing old and supporting yourself for a period of time on what you spent your lifetime earning, and then simply returning to dust.

Go back to the story I shared with you earlier when Jessie, our nurse practitioner, came in and just seemed a little off. I went to the nurse's station and told her to level with me. She did so by showing me the progression of the tumors and not the regression. She told me none of the treatments had had any efficacy and we were sliding down the hill quickly. Things were not looking good and we would most likely need a miracle going forward for earthly healing. My eyes filled with tears and Jessie hugged me. I just held on to her for what seemed like forever in the middle of the ward. She patted me on the back and helped pull me back together r... or so I thought.

I went back in the room and Julie took one look at me and knew exactly what I had been told. I really didn't have to say anything to her. She said, "They are growing, aren't they? The treatments are not working." All I could do was nod my head and the waterworks started to flow from my eyes. I collapsed onto the "bouch" and started to ugly cry. When I finally picked my head up, while still bawling, I looked over at my bride expecting to see the same thing. But I didn't. She was resting comfortably in the bed and she had this calmness about her. There was no visible stress in her face and her eyes had a little gleam in them. I was confused. I had just told her that the treatments were not working. Nothing we had done to date had had any medical success. We were staring down the barrel of her mortality. How much time would we have left together? Were we counting months, days or minutes left that we would share together? Were we running out of opportunities to build more memories?

When I pulled myself together, I said, "Did you hear what I just told you?" She nodded yes. I remember this whole thing as vividly as it was yesterday. I asked her, "Why are you not emotional?" I was literally falling apart. Her answer? "I am at peace because I feel Jesus' arms wrapped around me. He is telling me that I am alright. Everything is going as it should according to his plan. His hug is comforting, and I have never felt a peace like I feel right now. The only real negative feeling I have right now is I feel a little guilt for not being scared. I am worried about you and the kids and how things will work out for you if I don't get the earthly healing we have been seeking. But I know I will be alright. He is with me. I also know that even if I am not medically healed here on Earth, I will get my healing in Heaven. I have been promised that. And, I know that we will be together again very soon."

 Soon is a relative term. Five years, 50 years, 100 years - in the grand scheme it is really a blink of an eye. When we think about what a long time really is, what comes to mind? The earth has been around for about 4.5 Billion years. If I have lived to 90-ish, and it has been a long healthy life, the I know we will reunite in heaven in very short order. Looking back on this dialogue now, I am amazed at both her faith and her wisdom. At the time it did nothing to ease my grief or fear. I remember responding (actually blurting out), "Why don't I feel His arms around me? Why is He not comforting and hugging me? I need help, I need to feel Him and His presence as well." Julie, very calmly responded, "Come here and let me put my arms around you for now. Perhaps you are just not yet ready to feel his hug, or perhaps He feels you are not yet ready. But in the meantime, I know you are ready for my hugs and that will have to suffice for now."

I crawled up into her hospital bed, and the ugly cry began anew, but she held me tight and that felt good as well. The intensity of grief/fear mixed with the comforting embrace of my wife is something that will always be fresh in my mind. Always.

Looking back on that day, that hour of my life, I still tear up in amazement of the pure FAITH that she had. I have seen nothing like it before, nor have I seen anything close to it since.

To this day, I still struggle with my faith and perhaps that is why I don't think I have felt the embrace of Jesus around me, yet. I still hold onto my faith and don't give up on it because of what I saw that day, and one day my prayer is that I will be ready and receptive to feel that embrace from my God.

Pray for Healing - Monday, July 23, 2007 (Authored by Julie)

Today Brendan and I are going to go to the hospital to have some bloodwork done (of course) and to have the IV for tomorrow put in. I am drinking water like crazy to keep myself hydrated. (Gerald, I have a whopper of a "line" story for you later!)

I have decided that my best effort now needs to go into prayer. In the past my prayers have been for strength and wisdom, my family and the wisdom of the doctors. I didn't know that I could ask for, and receive, healing. I mean, aren't we taught that God knows his plan for us from the beginning ... from our time in the womb? If that is so, isn't it a futile action to pray for something like healing? At least, that was my thought process. In fact, I brought that up to Tom and Nancy (prayer mentors for Brendan and I) ... you may know Nancy from Kendall's baptism. She is one of her Godparents.

I gave Tom and Nancy my thoughts on prayer for healing and I was surprised ... their take is that with enough fervor and honesty our prayers can change God's mind.

A few people have posted, or emailed directly, instances of someone with terminal Cancer who miraculously recovered ... people with only months to live. I think about those people ... how did THEY pray? What did THEY tell God?

One of the blogs I have on our blogroll is Jaymun's Journey. Jaymun is a little boy Kendall's age who was born with Cancer. Right out of the womb, he had Cancer. I followed his fight closely. His parents posted daily about his condition, the hardships on their other children and the stresses they face. Jaymun was going through his tough times about the same time I was going through chemo myself. There was one night in particular that seemed crucial. Jaymun's health was spiraling and his little body was not doing the things it needed to keep fighting. His Dad posted a calling for prayers. He likened ... well, here is the statement that inspired me so much ...

> *"And I remembered a story from the Old Testament. It was about Moses standing on a hill praying for his people as they were fighting a battle against a treacherous tribe of bandits. Moses was holding his arms up in the air while he prayed. His people were driving the bandits back. Then Moses got tired and he lowered his arms. Then the bandits made a comeback. Moses raised his arms again and began to pray. Sure enough - the bandits fell back. He couldn't afford to let his arms drop when the fight was that crucial.*
>
> *Now ... for me, the beautiful picture here is not Moses on a hill with arms raised. It is his two friends*

*standing with him on
the hill ... each holding
up one of his arms ...
so Moses could pray
through - until God
helped drive away
EVERY LAST BANDIT."*

-Jaymun's Dad

*I remember reading his post
that night and crying and
praying, praying and crying, for
a family I have never met and
whose suffering was SO much
more than mine. The next
morning the first thing I did was
check the blog ... did little
Jaymun make it through?!?!
Miraculously, yes. In fact, he
made it through ALL of his
Cancer treatments and now his
blog shows pictures of a happy,
healthy baby.*

*Even though his blog is more
about their personal lives now, I
like to go back and remember
how their prayer inspired me so
much and how I KNOW all those
people praying for him that
night MUST have made the
difference.*

*As the road gets longer, it gets
harder.*

About a week ago we had requested another appointment with Dr. Bedikian (primary Melanoma Oncologist) ... just to look at options and assess. Last Friday I had a phone call from my nurse at MDACC saying that Dr. Bedikian had an opening at 3:30 and could I make it? It was 3:00 at the time. I happened to be in the car, I turned it toward the hospital and went. Brendan was watching the kids and couldn't make it to the hospital in time and Dan was tied up in a meeting. It was my first time to go to an appointment alone. It was just a conversation I was needing, so I wasn't concerned.

While in the waiting room there were two other folks waiting. One I recognized. He had been in the "not-so-supportive-support-group meeting" with Brendan and me. I asked how he was doing, and he had GREAT news. He had actually just gotten an all clear and was back for a scan review. This piqued the curiosity of the OTHER woman in the room ... she had been fighting melanoma for 5 years. At first glance that might seem rough,

In my opinion there has to be something more
out there. Again, I am not here to tell you what
that is. It is between you and your beliefs. But I
am urging you, believe that there is something
guiding and driving us as humans. What are you
out if you believe in God or a Higher Power and
give it recognition, love, and do good things in

his name for other humans, and the world in general. In the end, what if he does not exist? I submit you are out nothing. In fact, you WIN anyway because you lived a life with purpose and made the world and others better in the short time you were here. However, think about what you will be out if you do not believe and live your life as suggested above. Again, I don't know what it will look like, but I would rather have a seat at the table and a room in Heaven than be sent to what I understand as the alternative.

I offer you this post from Easter 2007 for reflection.

> *Happy Belated Easter –*
> *Monday, April 09, 2007*
>
> *Happy belated Easter to our Army of supporters out there. I hope all of you enjoyed some quality family time together as well as some time to quietly reflect on the reason for the holiday.*
>
> *For me, it took a life altering event to take time to TRULY understand what Easter is all about. I always knew that Easter was the celebration of Jesus rising from the dead for our salvations. But I had never really reflected on the events and its importance. I had also

*never known that He was
sacrificed on the cross not only
for our sins and salvation, but
for our illnesses as well.*

*Therefore, on the Holiest of
Holidays, we turn this weight of
Cancer over to you Lord Jesus in
hopes that you will hold us
firmly in your hands and see us
through this dark and seemingly
endless tunnel. We know that
all things are possible for those
who believe and trust in you
and we know that this
"experience" is just a part of
your master plan for us.*

*I hope this post makes you stop
and think, if only for a few
minutes and that it doesn't take
an event similar to ours to spark
such reflection within yourself.*

YAY GOD!

-Brendan

Chapter 11

Dish preparation

You now have all of the ingredients to prepare a dish that will guarantee that you and/ or your loved one will BEAT Cancer. So how do you prepare the dish?

Pour all the ingredients in a large mixing bowl. Add them in no particular order. You just need to make sure they get added in the exact quantities that were specified. It is absolutely critical that you do not forget or skip any of the ingredients. They all play off each other and not only will the absence of one of the ingredients make the dish taste "off" but each ingredient omitted reduces my guarantee that you will BEAT Cancer with a resounding knock out!

Once all the ingredients have been added to the bowl, mix it all together thoroughly, making sure all the ingredients blend smoothly. As you stir, the dish should gain a firm consistency as the flavors chemically react with each other very similar to a no - bake cheesecake.

What does a perfect dish look and taste like? How will you know if you made it correctly?

Living Full Days – Tuesday, October 17, 2006

Under the blog post "Humor is Medicinal" my brother Derek referenced a speech by former

North Carolina *State basketball coach Jimmy Valvano in the comments section. If you are a sports fan, you have probably heard of him. If you have had Cancer or an intimate encounter with Cancer, there is a good chance you know of him. (The V Foundation is an organization he founded with ESPN to help fund Cancer research.) However, if none of the above apply, let me introduce you to him because I believe everybody who has been touched by Cancer should know about this man.*

Jimmy V, as he was known, was successful in everything he did. He was a star basketball player at Rutgers University. He was twice the Basketball Coach of the Year in his conference, had a winning coaching record, and was promoted to North Carolina State Athletic Director. His crowning achievement as a coach was in 1983 when he won a National Championship and led an over-achieving group of young men to a stunning victory over the talent - laden and number one team in the country, University of Houston

Cougars (Phi Slamma Jamma as they had been nicknamed). When he left North Carolina State he went into broadcasting and earned a Cable Ace Award.

However, what is mentioned above is not why I think you should know him. Jimmy V. was diagnosed with Cancer at the age of 46. He died one year later. During that one - year battle he lived his life with as much zeal and enthusiasm as he did for the first 46 years of his life. I still remember him running around the court hollering at the top of his lungs with arms raised above his head after the game - winning shot against my (at the time) beloved Cougars. He did not let Cancer define who he was or let it take away what he wanted to get out of life.

The essence of this spirit was captured in a speech he gave at the ESPY awards in 1993 and has come to be known as the "Don't Ever Give Up Speech." I encourage all of you to seek out this speech on the internet and watch it in its entirety. The speech is roughly 10 minutes long, so give yourself the time to watch it with your full attention. I promise you, you won't be sorry as he offers many valuable tips on how to live life. In my opinion, he did more in 10 minutes for people (especially those touched by Cancer), than some people do in a lifetime.

Having been touched firsthand by Cancer now, I find the following excerpt to be of particular importance and I think truer words could not be spoken.

> *"To me, there are three things we all should do every day. We should do this every day of our lives. Number one is laugh. You should laugh every day. Number two is think. You should spend some time in thought. And number three is, you should have your emotions moved to tears, could be happiness or joy. But think about it. If you*

*laugh, you think
and you cry, that's
a full day. That's a
heck of a day. You
do that seven days
a week, you're
going to have
something special."*

All three of these elements are found in the delivery of his speech.

Since I rediscovered my sense of humor a week and a half ago (thanks to Julie), I have been living VERY full days.

I make sure I find a reason to laugh each day, whether it be at myself or with family or friends. I laugh at some of the comments left on this blog. I call up my friends and "cut up" with them about things going on in my life or theirs. I play silly games with my kids or laugh at their "views on life" as only a young child can relate.

I spend some time in thought outside of work and /or everyday issues. I have started to keep a daily journal in addition to this blog where I document my day and my

musings. I think about my faith
and relationship with God and
what His master plan is for me
and my family.

And finally, not a day goes by
where my emotions are not
moved to the point of tears.
Admittedly they are not always
tears of happiness or joy and
are sometimes fueled by anxiety
over our current situation.
However, I have now found that
other things invoke this
physiological response. I look at
my children when they are
sleeping. I reflect on the
friendships and bond I have
built with my wife and mother
of those three beautiful
children. I think about my
parents and the support that
they always provide. I receive
emails and phone calls from my
brother, who despite his own
busy schedule at law school, is
spending whatever time he can
networking with his colleagues
and researching Melanoma to
help us battle this disease. I
think about my in-laws and
their acceptance of me into
their family from day one. I
think about the generous offers
of prayers and support in any

form from my friends and colleagues in addition to the "army" that has grown from them.

In spite of Cancer that is invading our lives right now … I am learning that I am very blessed and live "full days." And Jimmy V. was right … they are full days because I sleep like a rock each night!

-Brendan

PS … If you think God is not present at times and delivering a message to all of us, I offer you this … At the time Jimmy V. gave that speech, the Cancer had ravaged him physically to the point that he was so weak and he had to be carried onto the airplane to get to New York and pushed in a wheelchair into the auditorium. However, note that he walked to the podium, stood and delivered his speech without any assistance. He died a few short weeks later. In retrospect, I believe God gave him the sudden strength to deliver that message.

What you read above (and maybe you even watched the video) is exactly what the dish should look, taste and feel like!

Chapter 12

The Victory

My wife Julie claimed her VICTORY from Cancer on November 24, 2007. And not only did she claim this victory in this title bout, she kicked its ASS! She came into the ring at five feet and 4 inches tall and well, let's just say height weight proportionate … (I learned you never talk about a woman's weight!) against a Goliath that stood one hundred times her height and weight with an immeasurable reach. She gave Cancer a 13-month long ass kicking.

Now, so as not to mislead, she claimed her VICTORY in Heaven as a winner against Cancer on the date I just mentioned. While we did not receive the medical victory we were seeking, we received the most important VICTORY of all. The one that CCancer so desperately seeks. To terrorize you and cause you to stop living the moment you find out that it has taken up residence inside your body.

This woman never once gave up and fought that prick named Cancer from beginning to end. If you still doubt me, I offer you this short story …

If you look back at the calendar for the date that she passed you will find that November 24th of that year was the Saturday after Thanksgiving. Back up to the Wednesday before the holiday. She was scheduled for a chemo treatment that day. She was in a wheelchair at this time as tumors had attached to her spine and she had lesions in her brain effectively paralyzing her from the waist down. Getting her anywhere was a challenge but we were not going to let Cancer stop us from anything. We had an upstairs master bedroom, so I got her dressed, carried her to the stairs, helped her do her "scooch" move down the stairs, got her in her wheelchair, got her to the car and loaded her up. We got there at our scheduled appointment time which was somewhere around mid-day. But as so often happens at MDCCA we got delayed and delayed. We spent the day talking, surfing the internet, doing some of the puzzles that are laid out all over the waiting room tables and just trying to pass the time. We were finally called for the treatment administration at around 10 p.m. It was a slow drip and we did not complete it until around 2 a.m. We got home around 2:30 Thanksgiving morning and did the reverse routine mentioned earlier to get her upstairs and into bed.

We were scheduled to have Thanksgiving dinner at my sister-in-law's house about an hour and a half away in the Texas countryside. I made arrangements for my in-laws to take the kids out there early in the morning so we could get a little extra sleep and meet them later once we got moving around and could go through our routine yet again.

Later, we got moving and headed out to the country for Thanksgiving lunch, which coincidentally was Julie's favorite holiday and she loved the food. We had a great time driving and talking; the two of us never uttered a word about Cancer. It was not invited to this special day. Even though she had had a chemo treatment the night before that generally would affect her appetite she could not wait to get into the turkey and other fixings. She ate like she hadn't eaten in months and went back for seconds on a few things and even sampled some desserts. She did get a little tired at one point and asked to be taken to a back bedroom for a quick nap, but it was a very quick nap and she was back out with us sharing family time until it was time to go.

We decided to leave the kids with the in-laws and let them play out in the country for a day or two with their cousins and allow Julie (and myself) to catch up on some rest. The last chemo treatment she received was a particularly vicious concoction for her to take but we were praying that it would have the same effect on the Cancer.

We got home, and again went through our new routine. Wheelchair into the house, followed by me helping to pull her up the stairs and then carrying her to the bedroom. I got her situated in the bathroom so she could brush her teeth and go through her nightly routine. I then got her into her pajamas and into bed. We talked a little more and we said goodnight, with her saying, "I love you Brendan" and I responded in kind with "I love you too, Jules."

I laid there in bed and started to drift off when I heard her repeat to me, "I love you." I stirred from my semi-state of slumber and again repeated that I loved her too. Immediately she said it for a third time, and I (much to my regret afterward) said I loved her as well, but this time with a tiny bit of exhaustion. We then both fell asleep.

A short time later, I woke to a loud thud. I thought she had fallen out of bed and sprang to my feet asking what had happened. She said, "I was just getting up to go to the bathroom." I said, "What? You know I have to help you. Why didn't you wake me?" She asked, "Why would I do that, because I just had to go?" I replied, "Because you can't walk," which seemed to surprise her, which in turn surprised me. I then asked if she knew she had Cancer and she had no idea. I started asking her some other questions that were very basic to our family. How many kids do we have? What are their names? Where do we live? And so on. Some of the questions she got right, and she seemed annoyed that I would be asking such silly things. However, on several she replied with incorrect responses or gave nonsense answers. I had no idea what to do. I called some friends and explained what was going on. I put the phone on speaker and started my questions routine again so they could hear and to prove to myself that I wasn't going crazy as this was all very surreal to me. They heard her responses on speaker phone and told me to get her to the hospital right away.

I did just that, carrying her to the stairs, scooching her down the stairs and skipped the whole wheelchair thing altogether and carried her to the car.

When we got to the hospital, I parked the car in the emergency drop off area and rushed around the car to get her. I carried her in, frantically telling the intake personnel what was going on. They took her from me and put her in a wheelchair. They asked me to move the vehicle and return immediately to that very desk. When I returned, they were already taking her in for scans. When the scans were finished, I was able to spend some time holding her hand while the scans were reviewed and analyzed. Soon thereafter, the doctor returned and told me the bad news. The pressure was building in her brain and the lesions were blocking the ability for the fluid in her brain to naturally drain. She was going to go into a coma and pass soon.

As she was slipping into the coma, I called my in-laws and had them race the kids to the hospital. Easily a two-hour drive even in the middle of the night. The kids got there but Julie had lost her ability to respond. Each kid gave her a hug and in their own way said their goodbye to Mommy. She knew they were there as I could see a small smile on her lips and one tear in her eye. The kids left, and a few short hours later, surrounded by family she DEFEATED her Cancer by taking her rightful place in the house of the Lord.

I don't tell this story, to evoke sadness. I share this story to demonstrate just how hard this woman fought Cancer to the very end and continued to use the recipe in this book to steadily BEAT Cancer into a bloody pulp. WINNING against Cancer sometimes means you beat it medically and continue your Earthly life. Other times It means you win against it by not taking your Earthly life while you are here and fight like Hell against it medically while living everyday of your life as best as you can - enjoying what you have and the time that you have until you just flat don't have any more time.

Like I have said previously, any one of us can pass at any time. Car accidents, in-home accidents, other medical ailments, personal violence or any number of other things. We never know if today is our last. Cancer just gives you a potential timeline and terrorizes you into giving up on living life for whatever time it resides within your body. Tell it to go to Hell by eating a hearty bowlfull of this recipe each and every day and YOU WILL WIN. There will be no more, "He/ She lost her battle with Cancer." Get out of here with that noise. "He/ She WON their battle with Cancer and has taken their rightful place in heaven. He/ She left this world an absolute WINNER."

Epilogue

I know Julie is still with me. I see signs of it all the time. When we had to come to the conclusion that medical healing was a longshot for us, I told her that I would need to have some kind of sign from her that she was around and still with me. She said, "OK … We have three kids and one of our little things has always been three tugs of the ear to secretly say, 'I love you' in public places. When you see things in threes you will know I am around." I said OK. I got it.

The moment she passed, the first thing I notice was a flower arrangement someone had sent us sitting on the counter opposite me. In the middle of it was three sunflowers … sunflowers being one of her favorite flowers. I was grief stricken but I did have a brief smile on my face and silently I told her I was proud of her and how she BEAT Cancer and was comforted that the Cancer was now no longer a part of her being.

I started to see things in threes all over the place and suddenly I started waking up for about one solid week at 3:33 a.m. or randomly noticing the same time in the afternoon as my eyes were randomly drawn to a clock at that exact time. It still happens today but not as often as I think she knows that I do OK for the most part these days. But true to our deal, I still notice that time of day or night time and again or see other things in threes, just so that I know she is there.

Remember, just before we went to sleep that Thanksgiving night and completed our last conversation together? She told me she loved me three times. As I look back on that, she knew what was going to happen and she was prepping me for her messages in threes.

My Eulogy to her is themed with the number 3.

Thank You … Times 3

Thank you for saying "yes" almost 11 years ago. That one-word response simply made me the happiest and most fortunate man in God's Kingdom. It provided me not only a partner with whom to share my deepest feelings, my biggest fears, my greatest moments, and my lowest moments but it provided me with an eternal sense of security in that I was loved simply because I was Brendan. Regardless of what life threw at me, I knew that I would have your unmitigated support to get me through it.

Over the years, I have developed a personal philosophy of trying not to take myself too seriously and using humor to help get me though the ups and down of life. I often wondered if I would ever find someone to share my life with that would have a similar philosophy as well as a sense of humor that was similar to mine. Fortunately, I did. When you were diagnosed and we got over the initial shock (which for you was about 24 hours and me about 24 days), you leaned on your sense of humor to help you live out each day of your life by having fun. I documented on our blog how you approached the administration of your first round of chemotherapy. When the nurse entered the room, she flippantly asked, "How are you?" Without missing a beat, you responded, quite nonchalantly, "Well, I have a little bit of the Cancer today." I don't care who you are ... That's funny! I could go on and on with examples of your sense of humor.

Your acceptance of my marriage proposal allowed me to live with the most supportive partner one could ever ask for. If I enjoyed something or had my heart set on something you always supported me and found a way to make it happen even if it made your life more difficult or you had to sacrifice something you wanted or wanted to do. You were selfless to the extreme. Case in point, would be my love for basketball officiating. You were never a big sports fan, and quite frankly the game of basketball (which I grew up playing through college) was quite boring to you. Buy you knew I had a passion for officiating and always found a way to help me advance in the *officiating ranks. You accepted the fact thouGH you were a "basketball widow" from the months of late November through early February, because you knew it was important to me. In the offseason, you always made sure that the finances were in order for me to attend the many training clinics around the country as I have pursued my dream of moving up the officiating ladder. You never complained about being left with all three kids on a game night or a camp weekend (even though the past season you were battling Cancer) and in fact you insisted that I keep an aggressive schedule because you knew how fulfilling officing was to me outside of my family and professional life. You knew that it was my outlet and a chance for me to clear my head and do something I enjoyed ... You also never complained about all the checks that showed up in the mailbox through the course of those three and half months either!!! In fact, recently you made me reassure you that regardless of the outcome of our battle with Cancer, that I would find a way to continue to pursue my officiating goals. I promise you, baby, I will do that and will take comfort each time that I take the floor that you are right there with me ... helping me to make the right calls and handle the difficult coaches and situations.*

Not too long ago we were sitting around with Nancy (who more or less has become a spiritual advisor to us) reading some scripture and discussing our feeling and fears. It was one of the only times I saw a chink in your armor, and you broke down. You were so concerned about what this battle was doing to me and made the statement to the effect, "I am so sorry for Brendan. This is so tough on him and had he known that this battle was in his future, he probably never would have chosen this path." I have told you three times since that statement, once later that night, once a few weeks later during a late night at MDACC and one last time just before you passed away. I would choose this very path knowing that would happen every day of the week and twice on Sundays because the short time we had together on this earth was more than worth the pain and suffering that I am experiencing right now losing my best friend.

Thank you for providing me with three beautiful and loving children, who each and every day going forward will remind me of the 11 plus years we spent together ... a year or so of dating and 10 years and nine days of marriage. You were the perfect mother ... patient yet stern, loving, selfless and dedicated. The list of positive adjectives is endless. The kids always came first to you and you always made sure that they knew they were loved as you always had a cabinet full of activities for them to do on rainy days and took them on outdoor adventures on sunny days. You always made sure that they were healthy and comforted them when they were sick or injured. You were so in tune with them, that you could immediately sense when they had an ear infection, while I would just assume that they were just whining and needed to "suck it up." I hope and pray that over the years going forward I can become half the parent to those kids that you have been. I am far less equipped in terms of parental aptitude to raise these kids than you ever were.

My commitment to you is that I will do everything I can to raise our kids as you would have wanted and make you proud. My goal is to have you smiling down from Heaven upon them as they grow and mature and become the successful individuals that you surely would have turned them into had God not had other plans for you.

Julie, these kids will "KNOW" their mother. I will speak of you every day to them. I am already advising them that they can talk to you about anything ... their fears, their sadness, their joys, successes, etc. and that you will always hear them and be with them. Even though you will not be able to answer them in an audible voice, I have assured them that you will answer them by influencing their thoughts and actions and leaving them subtle signs that you are by their sides and have not abandoned them, but rather have gone to a place where you can be with each of them always, instead of only when you were physically with them here on Earth.

Thank you, Julie, for being my hero and inspiration as well as demonstrating to countless many how to live each and every day with strength, confidence and FAITH in the Father Almighty. I mentioned earlier, after you were diagnosed it took you about 24 hours to pick yourself up by the bootstraps and dig your heels in to fight this insidious disease. Each and every time we received a setback and we were knocked to our knees you quickly regained your strength and placed our faith in Jesus that this was just a mere setback. You analyzed what our options going forward would be, you prayed over them, made a decision and went forward knowing that this time it was going to produce the needed results. Obviously, we did not receive the results we were hoping for in terms of beating the Cancer here on Earth, but I take comfort in knowing that you BEAT the

Cancer and are now reaping the rewards of your unwavering faith in the Kingdom of God. You did BEAT Cancer as I told you in the hospital shortly before Jesus came to escort you to your home in Heaven. I believe that you did fulfill your goal in BEATING Cancer. You did not lose. For the only way to lose to Cancer is to allow it to steal your spirit, your Faith and your motivation to live. Cancer can be beat in two ways, either by earthly medicine mixed with Faith in Jesus Christ or by living your life each day as Jesus would have wanted you to with unwavering strength, faith and courage and taking your rightful place in Heaven. The Cancer is dead, and you are alive and well in the Kingdom of the Lord finally free of this awful disease.

Through our blog you were able to reach out to so many people and positively influence how they lived their life as well as quite possibly save some lives in the process - both physically and spiritually. I have been told by many people that due to your candor and honesty about how your disease developed, they have had their skin screened and, in some cases, had "suspicious" moles removed or moles that were in the early stages of melanoma removed. You have saved people spiritually as well. I am atop that list as I had allowed my Faith in God to erode. I know your good friends have acknowledged that their spiritual life has been renewed. This is just two immediate examples, but if you read the blog you will see hundreds if not thousands of people, who have found God, returned to God or have strengthened their relationship with Him. And for that, you have truly done God's work in bringing Faith into many lives here on earth.

You should have noticed a theme in the Eulogy. I thanked my dearest Julie three times over and told her three times that I would have married her knowing that our time would be short on three separate occasions, as the number three is the cornerstone of our relationship.

Shortly after we were married, we developed a non-verbal signal to express our love for each other. We called it "Two Tugs" as we would gently tug on each other's ear twice to simply say "I Love You". As we were drifting off to sleep, we might exchange "Two Tugs" or if we were in a public place where we may not want to verbalize the message we would exchange "Two Tugs." However, you decided that since we now have three wonderful children, the number should be changed to three. We would now exchange "Three Tugs" or give each other kisses in threes.

I have trouble with things that I cannot see or touch. When we recently discovered that our chances of defeating Cancer here on Earth were waning, I found myself in deep despair. I told Julie, that I HAD to know that she was with me. That she would have to find a way to show me a tangible sign and "speak" to me so that I would know without a doubt that she was by my side and guiding me through life as my Guardian Angel. She said, "Our sign will be the number three. When you see or experience things in groups of three you will know that I am with you and by your side." This gave me some comfort.

Julie, I know you have already spoken to me on THREE different occasions since you departed this Earthly life. When we got to the hospital and we learned that your death was imminent. I immediately put in a call to our Church. Father Tran got there as soon as he could Friday morning to deliver Last Rites. Later that evening, Father Mike arrived and prayed over you that you would be comforted by the Father, that your pain would be eliminated, and that your anxiety would be non-existent as the Father made his final preparations for your arrival in His Kingdom. Father Dan was out of town and did not arrive until late Saturday evening. As he was praying over you, Jesus came and took your hand from mine and carried you to Heaven. You left to be with the Father upon the arrival of the third priest from our church.

When I finally realized you had ascended to Heaven, one of the first things I notice was the flower arrangement across the room on the counter that some of our friends had sent to us. In the middle of the bouquet, were three wonderfully vivid sunflowers … As you loved sunflowers, I knew it was you speaking to me and letting me know that you were present with me and comforting me as I grieved uncontrollably. It gave me comfort.

Lastly, when I attended the Life Teen mass this weekend, the gospel was Luke 23:35-45. It speaks of Jesus being crucified with two other criminals … totaling three simultaneous crucifixions at the time of Christ's death. The final verse in the Gospel reads, "Jesus answered him, 'I tell you the truth today you will be with me in paradise."

You were speaking to me. As the third event tells me in the final verse of the Gospel … you are with him today in paradise.

Until we meet again in person in paradise know that …

I LOVE YOU JULIE

I LOVE YOU JULIE

I LOVE YOU JULIE

Before letting this recipe cool and closing the chapters on this book, I want to share one final story. It was a post in my blog and maybe the final entry, but somehow it did not get reprinted in the book when the website was taken down, so I will have to recount the story from memory and this is not hard for me to do; I have told the story many times and the powerful nature of the story itself keeps it real. It is my personal testimony.

If everything I have written thus far doesn't convince you that this recipe will work to guarantee victory against Cancer one way or the other, I leave you with this ...

Every year Julie would buy me a Valentine's Day card and leave a brief message in the card for me. She would leave these cards for me in various places where I would stumble across them at differing parts of the day. Sometimes they were left by toothbrush and razor. Sometimes they were left by the coffee pot. I remember another time where it was found on the dashboard of my truck. However, one year, a few years before she passed, she put one in my briefcase. I did not find it until I got to work.

A few days before the Valentine's Day after she passed, I was feeling really down and depressed. I was sitting in the living room with my mom with tears in my eyes and was lamenting that this was the first time in eleven years that I would not be finding a Valentine's Day card from Julie. My mom just listened, gave me a hug and did her best to console me.

I went to work on Valentine's Day and knew I had to leave work early because I had a function with one of the kids shortly after school, so I was under the gun to get things done. About mid-day I got a call from a former administrative assistant in a department I used to work in for my company. I had changed offices several times since then and was working in a new group. Several people had occupied my old office since I had vacated it. She said I needed to come see her. I told her that I could not make it that day but would come by the next morning. She insisted that I make time that day and come by. It was important and would not take long, so I reluctantly agreed.

When I got there, she said, "I was cleaning out the office you formerly occupied and I found this manila folder and just grabbed it thinking it was empty but something fell to the floor." She opened the envelope and showed me what it was that fell to the floor. It was the Valentine's card that she put in my briefcase a few years before. I teared up as I did get my Valentine's Day card from her that first Valentine's Day without her. But even more special and appropriate was the message of the card. The card is in the shape of a house. It reads:

Front: For my Husband

Inside: Home is being happy in the everyday things … Home is all the Love we share. Home is you and me. Happy Valentine's Day

In her own pen: I Love Being Home! All my love, Julie

Several years ago, the card had one meaning. When I got the card the Valentine's Day after her passing, the card had a whole new meaning. She was happy being *home* in Heaven but was still with me and we still shared the same love … Her and me. I think that it is also interesting to note the references in the card that speak directly to the ingredients in this "recipe." Interesting isn't it?

Later I found a notebook of instructions in my desk that she left me. In there were instructions and tips on raising the kids, how and where to buy furniture and many other things. But the longest entry was to not be afraid and find love again and remarry if the situation was right.

I did just that in 2012 and am now remarried to a wonderful lady that has taken on me and all my flaws. She has taken on my children as her own despite joining me with two of her own. We share a love that is strong and unique in and of itself. Julie is a part of my life forever, and Carrie accepts that. But she needs to know that even though we share a similar love that has its own uniqueness that is not the same as the relationship I had with Julie, but nonetheless is just as special to me in its own individual way. I love you Carrie and all you have done for me and my children.

Ladies and Gentlemen, this concludes the recipe for kicking Cancer's Ass. Follow it to the tee and you will always WIN THE WAR WITH CANCER. That is a guarantee! The guarantee does not always mean Earthly healing, but it does mean WINNING one way or the other. Everyone is a Winner if they make the conscience choice to be a WINNER.